DO NO HARM
(except to you)

A Story of Crohn's Disease, survival, malpractice and defiance

Ethan Moore

I would like to give a special thanks to the doctors at the Cedars-Sinai IBD Center for keeping me alive when no one else would, and absolutely no thanks to a buttload of other people.

I'm still alive, so obviously it could have been worse. Others have had things worse, but their graves are silent. Other people haven't been as lucky as me in certain ways. My life has been like I'm flying off the cliff in one moment and back on the road in the next seen, it makes no sense, but it doesn't have to make sense. I just know it happens. I also know that one day it won't happen anymore. Others haven't been so lucky. Whenever things would reach the point when survival seemed impossible, I could at least intermittently make it back to Cedars-Sinai for at least short times, where there were the only doctors to actually try to save me. That was only intermittently, and the rest of the time I was on my own with a deadly problem(s). It would be at the last moment when somehow things would work out and I would get enough care to get me back functioning, until I would end up somewhere else. My luck wasn't just with health, although many incidents can't be separated from it. When a nutcase gunman opened fire, was is a random change in air density or a small bug sneezing on a blade of grass and setting off an improbable chain reaction that the bullet didn't have the right lead angle? Who knows, but I know because of the other victims that he had no lack of ability, which is no fault of those less lucky. I won't know what happened in my case, and all I know is that if that bullet came at me an inch over I would have lost much more than a windshield. Some people don't get those last moment miracles, or even have options open up, ever, no how desperate they get trying to find someone who will save them, or even care if they live or die. On the other hand, some people are able to find emotional and spiritual support systems which were denied to me. It isn't enough for resources to exist somewhere, they have to be available to those who need them, or somehow made available. Even if someone can work out a way to get care covered, people can still have logistical matters than can't always be overcome, and people are still stuck with whatever is available in their location. There are other factors in whether someone lives or dies. Look at the outcome statistics when things like race or poverty get involved. I also started with some tools in my box others didn't get. Some people can obviously point to worse things that they went through and survived, and I haven't been through the worst. We need to hear their voices. Someone has to say something.

What does it take for healing to begin?

In the television show The Simpsons, there is a character by the name of Dr. Nick Riviera. A general positive disposition and good bedside manner don't make up for lack of knowledge. He may have found his doctorate in a cereal box, and his board certification may not be worth the paper it's printed on even counting for inflation (in cartridges are expensive these days.) Known for being inept, it is possible to laugh at the failures of such a character, until one meets a real doctor with serious problems. Imagine if there were entire hospitals filled with Dr. Nick's siblings and cousins. There was one thing about him which deserved respect, though. To save Homer Simpson's life, Dr. Nick was willing to set aside the hubris of rank and title and listened to an 8 year old girl who know what needed to be done and guided him through the surgery that he wasn't qualified to perform.

And then there is real life. What is worse than Dr. Nick? When malice and deliberate harm enter the picture on top of stupidity.

Things aren't happening in a vacuum. There is more to a disease than the physical effects. A disease is a matter that is social, emotional, mental and spiritual with no part of life that isn't affected in some way and work combine to make the disease what it is. This fact influences both the coping and the treatment. It is important to have a support system, although such does not exist for everyone. Sometimes the physical part of the disease is the lesser part. Sometimes the worse disease is not the one inside one's body, but the one surrounding the person.

This is not in any way a comprehensive story of my life. There are many more experiences which could be included, but I have included the experiences which relate to certain points which are the focus of this work. There are other books which can and should be written on a number of subjects brought up in this work, and a number of rabbit holes these talking points could go down. The experiences mentions, although there are many more, are mentioned to make certain points. Even though there are religious references, due to that being part of my experience, I will limit such to what is directly relevant to the experience.

This being about my experiences, I can't speak very kindly about some segments of society, and I can't apologize for that without becoming a liar. Maybe other people have had different experiences with them, but that doesn't change what they did to me. Some people experience the best of certain groups, I experienced the worst of those groups.

So, when does healing begin? Healing begins after survival.

Most of my blood went missing, again

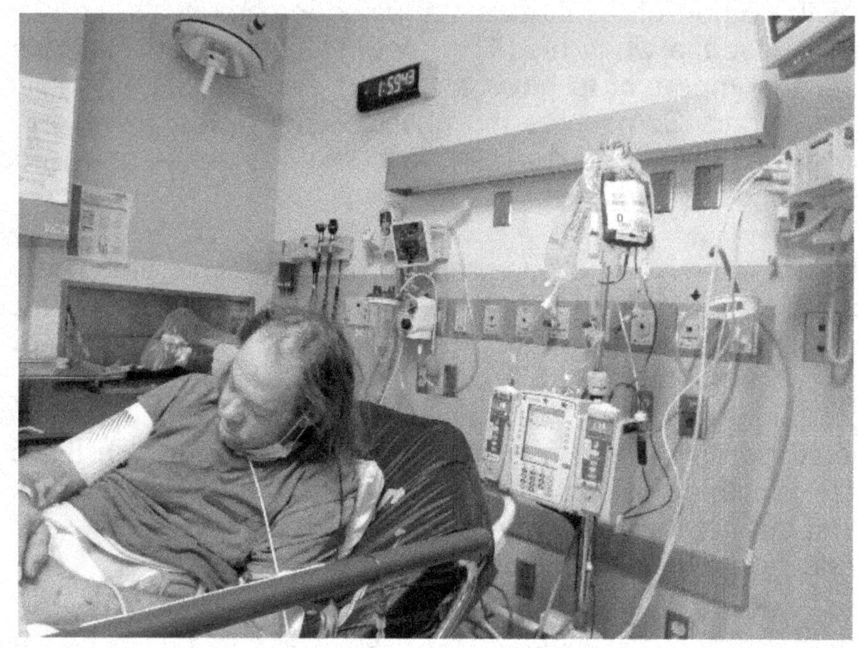

1

A long time ago, I had a dream that I called the dream of the Device. In that dream, I was taken to a mental hospital and they had me watch a patient through a two-way mirror. The patient had a small object and was making adjustments to this device which they had constructed. It was implied that the patient was sent there because of inventing this device. It was considered to be imaginary, and the doctors were trying to get that person to abandon the device. The person would not give up what they had built, and continued to faithfully work on it in spite of the damage to their life inflicted by those who don't understand, or even want to understand.

The doctors talked to me about the device, which no one knew the purpose of. They told me that it isn't real and can't do anything, merely because they didn't know what it does. None of those doctors even bothered to ask the patient any questions about their creation.

Then the patient turned on the device. It began spinning and doing something. The doctors continued staring at the scene, while telling me that what was happening in that room wasn't actually happening at all. When someone is designated crazy for pursuing their vision, all things in relation to that person are then automatically judged to be crazy and confirmation bias takes priority over observable facts.

The device kept working, moving faster and faster with each spin. I could clearly see it was doing something. I tried to get the doctors to look at it moving. Here was proof that it was something real, and not just a figment of imagination. I just didn't know what it was doing or why it was built. I don't have to be able to explain it to be able to see it working. The doctors denied that it was doing anything. No one would listen to me. I'm not the one with a fancy piece of paper on the wall saying that I know more than everyone else and granting the power to destroy lives. I'm just another person who has to suffer for what someone else doesn't understand or even want to. Understanding takes looking at facts for what they are even if one doesn't like those facts, and a willingness to set aside any preconceived concepts which do not fit the facts, no matter how inconvenient.

Those doctors kept staring right at the facts. They then declared that the case was hopeless, since the patient would not give up on the devise that the doctors simply didn't want to exist. It is easier for many people to deny rather than change. One may pretend that something doesn't exist, but that will never make it go away.

Even though I was an observer in this dream, I had lived what it symbolized. It never ended. I was voiceless, since nothing I said mattered. It can be devastating to be caught up in someone's game. I've had to fight for every day I'm alive, beginning when I was seven, while being a pawn in the game of conceit. I have still been lucky in a way. Other people have these problems too. If I had been from one of the marginalized groups in America, there would have been zero chance of surviving the harm done to me by so many.

Part of living with this problem is dealing with people who don't or won't accept a reality that they are not going through. I have even had doctors mock my pain. Even more nurses have, with contempt of others seemingly part of their job. Only at Cedars-Sinai have things not followed that pattern.

My life depends on holding on to my device. I can't let anyone take away what I have. The device is my life. One day I might even understand this device and why it exists, but that isn't necessary for it to work. I do what must be done, no matter what opposition I have for not playing the game right. I know what it is like to even have family order me to give up and let myself die. That was literal, and coming from my own mother, and others, who pretend to do so because they supposedly care about me enough to want me dead. The disease can take much away. But that is a physical matter. There is an even worse disease which surrounds me, existing not in my intestines, but in the hearts of the people who can destroy both body and soul. And they have tried.

So, what is healing, anyway?

2

It began when I was seven, later in 1981. It began with the pain. This made things difficult. I wasn't believed. It was said that I was faking it to get out of a particular class at school, since the pain would occur at the same time of the morning. I will admit that I hated school. Eventually, someone though that I might not be faking curled in a ball on the floor screaming and puking. It took a while of that, though, so I wasn't checked by a doctor and given a diagnosis until 1982 when I was eight.

Even with a diagnosis of Crohn's disease, it was still said to be all in my head. The treatment I was given and an ant-acid and to go see a counselor. That didn't fix the problem, and the gaslighting didn't work either. Counseling sessions consisted of the counselor interrogating me like a criminal, and repeatedly demanding that I confess to some secret that was not even there- "What are you hiding?" repeated over and over again through every session, never once did I receive an acknowledgement that maybe I am sick and that is what is interfering in my life.

Eventually, since the Gestapo was unable to break me and get me to spill my alleged secrets, someone decided to maybe give medication a try. The only real one available at that time to treat something which was still a complete mystery to the medical world was prednisone. It at least slowed down the problem. I also created other problem, and they didn't want to put me on an effective dose at that age. Prednisone treatment ended up lasting 20 something years. I ended up half a foot shorter than other men in my family, and gave me bad teeth and bird bones, with my skeleton being more decorative than structural. It was unfortunate that I began treatment at Kaiser.

With crippling pain lasting hours to days at a time, puking, and uncontrollable diarrhea, it was hard to pursue things in life. It wasn't just that, though. The social effects were worse than any emotional effects, and the physical, emotional, social and spiritual all work together to produce the experience of this problem. The emotional effects are in my control, the social effects are what is inflicted on me by the choice of others. It was hard to participate in things. People found it easier to just keep me at a distance rather than learning about my problem. It became too great of a burden to continue playing the trumpet in the school band, since the practice tended to fall on a bad time of day. Sports could be hard, and with the malnutrition and the exhaustion from the pain that comes with Crohn's disease physical activity was difficult at times.

People knew something was different about me. It was easy enough to see that something is wrong. People didn't understand what I was going through, and that included children and adults. People somehow got the idea that I have to be treated a certain way, instead of just treating me like a normal person who just has a problem. I didn't expect (or receive) special treatment from people. It made things awkward. People didn't want to violate some social expectation, so they found it easier to just not have anything to do with me. The sad thing is that it wasn't my disease taking everything away, but the lack of understanding, or even a willingness to understand. There were a few friends, but it was impossible to become really close to people who don't want me close.

There were also double standards to face, when your problem is on the inside and not being waved like a flag to the world to see. I found out how I am only supposed to exist to appease people. There was more going on here. The self-appointed leader of the group of "friends" showed narcissistic behaviors that made me wonder why I even tried to have a friendship with him, or with any of them since they all just back him up in everything. One fact of all narcissists is that they back other narcissists up against a victim. I got to see things from another angle once when some kids I was trying to be friends with were visited by another kid with two missing fingers. They were trying to appease him however they could (and they weren't about to try applying that to my case with my invisible internal illness). That boy with the two missing fingers expected such treatment and that was what he got. He demanded to be given priority over everyone there. He had apparently been treated with such privilege, since he had a problem that was visible and he could milk for everything he could get, that he was one of the most entitle people I have ever met, and one of the more hostile ones too. He demanded such treatment from me, and I stood my ground against his raging tantrums, although only by silence. I didn't say anything to him or attack him for his behavior, which I felt needed some understanding to work through, since I could see where it was coming from, and he was as much a victim of it by the people around. The person I had to speak out against was the head narcissist who was also shouting commands to me, like he had been shouting to the others of the group, only I was the one who didn't bow down to him. I was then kicked out of the group for not playing the game right. Appeasing a dictator is NEVER a sign of caring or empathy, and is actually the opposite. But that one boy was only a symptom of a problem, not the only one there and *his* behavior, as unpleasant as it was, was not even the worst problem going on there. The reality I saw was that I was expected to appease *them*. They were the real dictators, and what was going on was abuse by proxy, using that boy to express their hatred of me, until it became direct from them. Could they really not see what was happening. Of course they could, but can't admit, since then they would have to admit that they were the ones encouraging destructive behavior and were part of the reason it was happening. I admitted not liking his behavior, and they told me that I don't like him because he has missing fingers, but that of course was only after I had stood up to them and they were seeking excuses. It wasn't possible to explain what hypocrisy is to kids, and they wouldn't listen to my explanation of why I objected to being treated like that by that boy. They expected me to treat that boy as someone different, while claiming that *they* were the ones treating him as a normal kid. I was treating him as a regular person, and they were the ones treating him different. I'm not saying that missing fingers is not a problem, but the worse disease was outside both me and that boy, making the experience of the disability a type of monster it never had to become. I wanted to be treated as a human being, without some double standard making everything a joke. It never occurs to people that maybe I would like to be treated with the same respect everyone demands from me. Maybe I would have liked to be a human being. Just because you can't see something from the outside doesn't mean it isn't there, but I never asked for special treatment. I had only tried to get acceptance, like I'm a person or something. It wouldn't have mattered anyway, since my difference apparently only deserved hatred and isolation.

Part of the irony was that isolation and exclusion were what they were giving to that boy, only in a different way, since they were making him as different from them as they could, but with a different excuse than what they used to exclude me. My "crime" was that I, as an inferior, stood up for myself against bullies.

I also overheard a conversation among that group (I lived next door) where they were talking about me and my pain sensitivity. It was another reason for them to have nothing to do with me, since I would scream out in pain so much. I was disappointed that they wouldn't acknowledge that I was already in severe pain, even though they knew about my problem, and it didn't take much to push it over the edge. Obviously people in society want their sick people completely disabled, like they were doing to destroy any chance the boy with the missing fingers would have at learning to be a member of society, since that would be less of a threat to their egos than someone working to overcome a serious problem they don't have to face. With me they won't be happy until they see a gravestone, and that is actually literal. The boy had a problem on the outside, so they worked to destroy him inside. My problem was inside, so they felt the need to attack me, even with me having to defend myself physically against half a dozen of them on one occasion. And, that occasion was simply a continuation of the one just discussed, and it was sparked by another person on my street showing interest in being my friend, and I was friendly in return. How dare someone they ostracized reach out to someone who actually wanted to be my friend! I turned out to not be as weak as they had told me I am, and they certainly must have sensed that if they felt it necessary to go 6 on one, especially since they still didn't take me down. Who are the weak ones? Did they think I was going to respect them for that? It is always open season on someone with a major problem in a predatory society, and we learn to survive. I can't say I felt betrayed, since I already know how they viewed me. I got used to being alone, and preferred to be alone. My real friends were trees, which always accept people for who they are, and they also never pretend to be what they are not. The trees also never betray someone. The truth was that I did feel bad that he had lost two fingers, and I can't say I know what it is like to lose fingers, but I do know what discrimination for a disability is like. I may not know that particular problem, but I know what it is like to have things taken away. I know what it is like to have limitations which placed many normal experiences outside of possibility. It could have become a moment of solidarity, but that was not what people wanted from their cripples, and they were sure to keep it from happening. No one sees me fighting for every day I'm alive. That doesn't leave much energy for much else. But, that doesn't mean that I can accept what was done to me, and having a problem does not mean that they can just bash me down into submission, even literally. My disease was an excuse, not the real problem.

It didn't work. I saw that they were dangerous and that I would have to be much more cautious around them. Since they were on my street, that was hard to avoid completely. That doesn't mean that I didn't have friends there, just not any in that clique.

If it was just bullying and hatred, I would have nothing to complain about compared to "normal" childhood. Other people go through much worse stuff than I mentioned, and people have had to face murder, particularly in certain demographics and locations. I had to face that too, some of which was directly related to my being sick. My luck shield was with me on those occasions. Others have not been so lucky, through no fault of their own. I can't take credit for surviving things. I can't explain why there was a single barely hand sized weed a just the right spot that actually held my weight that kept me from falling 100 feet when I slipped over a cliff. Sometimes it seems that the Grim Reaper is out taking a leak so often he really should get his prostate checked. Or maybe I have *Other* friends outside the scope of this book.

It wasn't just kids being stupid and immature, or that they were even the worst problem. All of them were actually just doing what their parents told them to do to me. Adults just considered me a problem child, although I was really good at following rules. *The device keeps spinning, people keep denying.* Being in crippling pain which the women who have Crohn's disease say it is worse than childbirth (women don't have a complete monopoly on pain) was not considered a valid reason for not sitting up straight and singing at the church. For some reason it is the most narcissistic people who demand someone sing, and they bring down all the hellfire and damnation they can muster if they don't get what they demand. I learned to not sing, and I won't sing at the command of devils.

There was every excuse for why I had to be isolated and not even allowed to participate in many activities. The idea that I might be sick was not one of those reasons. It is true that I couldn't share everything going on. Exposing a weakness was much worse than keeping it to myself. I couldn't just spend the night at a friend's house, since the diarrhea complicated things, and I would have to leave without giving anyone an indication why. Boy Scout stuff was often out of the question, and I was considered just lazy and a failure for not advancing as fast as those able to participate. Then the accusations began that I was a drug addict, and therefore a threat to others. Talking about Crohn's disease made no difference, and they all knew I had even had a surgery for it. To them I was just faking it. If it wasn't drugs (they never told me what drug they were accusing me of using) then the gaslighting would continue, with the adults trying to convince me that I don't have a physical problem and I am making it up because I must be severely depressed. I observed patterns, and it was easy to trace these lies back to my mother. Already having a bowel resection was somehow no proof. My mother knew the truth, but was spreading these lies to isolate me. It was effective among the dumbasses, and the intent was to cause me to give up.

And then there were doctors, or one in particular at that time. I got the impression, from the number of pediatricians I have met, that one has to fail a test to become one, and that includes ones I had met personally besides the ones I met professionally. I won't apologize for that any more than they are ever going to apologize to me for what they did to me. Pediatricians have a high percentage of narcissists, since narcissists go after those unable to fight back. It was bad enough going through what is the same as Munchausen Syndrome by proxy (my mother is actually a narcissist but they do the same things for the same reasons) but having a doctor jump on board with the gaslighting and sabotage of my life was bad too. I had disease pop up in my stomach. I had pain in my stomach from it which felt different from the bad spots in my intestine. This pediatrician tried to convince me that there was nothing wrong. I eventually got an endoscopy, and since they weren't into knocking people out for stuff back then, I had asked before the procedure if I could look through the scope also. At the end of the test, the doctor showed me the sore in my stomach through the scope. It was there like I said. The pediatrician afterward said that the test found nothing, and tried to convince me that I was wrong and there was actually nothing there and I have no disease. I needed a letter from the doctor for the school, since I was in too much pain, with anemia and malnutrition with it, for fully participating in PE. One day I was called into the vice principal's office. He showed me the letter from the doctor. The letter said that I am pretending to be sick for attention and there is nothing wrong with me. The letter instructed the school to "humor" me and go along with it anyway. This was after a bowel resection. It was easy enough to pull my shirt up and show the surgical scar. Did I fake the surgery? I refused to see that pediatrician, or any other one after that. I had been betrayed by the medical profession, again. That was only to prevent me from getting help, and it isn't just kids who are predators pouncing on anyone with a perceived weakness.

The school before that was a bigger problem. It was a Baptist school. All the same problems existed there as elsewhere, with some additional ones. It was more isolating than out in the general population, and I got to learn about absolute hatred. They added to my existing problems the problem of having to listen to them call for the extermination of people of my faith. Threats were constant. I complained, and tried to resolve things through normal channels, where they engaged in victim blaming. Even though they knew what was going on (an approved of it) they determined that I must be the problem, instead of protecting me from harm and holding people accountable they said I had to see a counselor. I went to a few sessions in that summer, with that Baptist counselor trying to convince me that there was nothing bad about what they were doing to me. That counselor tried to convinced me that I was the problem and I need to accept how I am treated and stop trying to say that what they are doing is wrong. How dare I try to protect myself from what sure seemed to me to be godless savages. (It was only many years later when I was no longer in Ridgecrest that I met other Baptists who didn't treat people like that. Ridgecrest is a city of extremes, and the problem was not limited to Baptists there. The problem was across the whole board in that town, and not limited to one group. What happened with that congregation happened because they were following their pastor's hatred, and I later found that other pastors and their congregations are not like that). I was told to accept what was being done to me, the point being that I deserved the abuse. Apparently, talking about exterminating people was OK as long as it is people like me and those of my faith they want dead. The bones of my ancestors are scattered across the plains from trying to escape murder. I fixed the problem. I refused to see that counselor and I refused to return to that school. Problem solved. They would just have to hate someone else. I had no friends there and did not even desire to have anything to do with them.

My second high school, which I transferred to in 11th grade, was different. Unfortunately it also added fuel to certain accusations. It was a special school for students who can't make it in a regular school. It had a reputation of being for drug addicts and pregnant girls. I found it different. There were no more drug addicts than at the other school. People treated eachother with noticeable respect. Everyone there had a problem, and everyone knew it or they wouldn't be there. The students there had no need for pretending and accepted people as they are. I enjoyed being around them. I was a part of a group, yet this group existed due to the isolation and contempt they all experience from people who couldn't understand what they were going through. They were going through bad stuff, and stuff best not shared. Even the teachers were treated awful by the school district, and there was a constant threat of the school being closed down. There was a severe lack of funding. Students were on their own. The teachers were not invited to district meetings. They planted the landscape and built a gazebo, and they took pride in the lawn, and anyone stepping on the lawn would be yelled at by every student around "Get off the grass!" The lawn was the pride of the students, the visible accomplishment of their determination to succeed in the face of opposition. These students with their disabilities could overcome their challenges. They had real strength which only comes through facing opposition, unlike those pretending to be something they aren't at the other schools, who only had a fake image of strength maintained by the fact that they never had to test it in a real problem. It is only the people who go through things who understand. I could be who I am and be safe around the Mesquite High School people. I might be willing to be around at least some of them now, but I have no contact with any of them.

3

There was an unexpected benefit from rejection: no peer pressure. Selling out to society and throwing away who I am (like my device) was never an option. The disease also allowed me to meet my wife. Consequences can be unpredictable sometimes, and I am far better off now than I would have been if I hadn't held on to who I am.

One recurring theme from counselors and others, is telling me that I must hate myself for being sick. I have tried to explain to the "professionals" that being sick is a circumstance I am in, and is not who I am, although it provided me much of the experience which shaped me and my life. There they went, looking for a problem to fix which wasn't there, never first checking to see that my "device" was working before declaring it broken. Why would I hate myself for something beyond my control, something I didn't choose? If I say that I am not depressed, why would they ignore my values and make up supposed proof that I must be lying. Those people obviously live in a very dark world that I want no part of, if that is the only way they perceive things. It gave me the impression that they must all hate themselves to assume hate is the only option for dealing with circumstances in life. And that even occurred with the counselor of the mandatory high school "self-esteem" class. I'm sure they hate themselves for a good reason, but that doesn't justify projection. My own mother, aware of what Crohn's disease does to a person, also continued the gaslighting nonstop, insisting that she knows this stuff because she took one introductory psychology course back in the sixties. She knows about the exhaustion which comes from intense daily pain and anemia, but still told me that fatigue is a symptom of depression and so that proves that I must be *clinically depressed*. That wasn't much of a course she took, if she wasn't taught that something can only be a symptom of depression if it is caused be depression and not something else like the chronic illness she knows I have.

The dumbasses also pitched in to try to reinforce the gaslighting. I had to face that stuff attending church also. Kind of like one instance of a man hinting that I was severely depressed, describing to me how you know someone is depressed because they look down. He was referencing an incident a couple days before that conversation when I was out for a walk around town and he drove by. I was looking down, but to call it depression is to ignore the fact that it was late in the day and I was facing the sun. Should I label *that* guy depressed because he was also trying to shade his eyes from the sun? By his own criteria, I can label him depressed. Here I am, like in a mental institution with my "device", but I am the one being stared at, and everyone thinks they are a psychiatrist and can somehow cure me of a problem that exists inside *their* heads. Confirmation bias is a very powerful weapon.

Oh yeah, and my problems also managed to bring me and my wife together. Long story, though. This disease is a trickster, popping up in every part of life for better or worse (mostly worse or whatever word they use for something beyond worse). Amy sent me a tape of her favorite songs and wrote a letter while I was in the hospital in 1992, but the tape had to wait until I got out. The batteries were going dead in a little tape player I had, and with the options of that tape, Suicidal Tendencies and Iron Maiden, I had to make a judgement call and I stand by my choice. I did listen to it when I got back home. Amy wasn't the only one who reached out to me at the hospital. The high school students all signed a number of cards, which I still have since I knew of their sincerity. Some young people at the church also sent some letters, but only because their leaders told them too. When I got out of the hospital, those young people were caring enough to go right back to pretending that I don't exist. Some different others reached out to me also, but there is no need to discuss *those* people.

It should seem odd, but appears to be normal, that one can't turn to religious people for emotional support and friendship when there is something wrong. The more positive response was the announcement at the church that they don't think that I would be able to survive this one, since if I was going to die, and almost did, complete with the near death experience, then they wouldn't have to continue making an effort to destroy me. The ones who are safe are hard to find. A noticeable effect at the church of me having another surgery for a problem they denied I have was that since there was an obvious reason for my problems they had to stop saying that I was a drug addict. So then they moved on to claiming that I was a *drug dealer*! I liked to play Hackysac, and they explained to me that it is only drug dealers who play that. The accusation predated that, they were just grasping any excuse they could to try to give credibility to their dishonesty, no matter how asinine. As one myth is replaced by another in the medical world, one lie is replaced by another in the general world. And here they are trying to convince me that *I'm* the one mentally ill!

So, nothing actually changed there. The trickster is good at shuffling cards to keep the game going long past its obvious bedtime. Another myth was busted. Being alone does not make someone lonely. I enjoyed wandering the desert alone and meditating. A spot of that desert then became what I called my Church, since I had a religion and no church surrounded by people who have a church and no religion. Very special experiences occurred in that desert which kept me going through the darkest moments of my life. I knew that I was in God's hands and I need not fear. So that certain crowd of people tried to take even that away from me, eventually even forcing me to leave Ridgecrest under threat of death from them. Can you imagine going to church and getting death threats right there? How Christ-like of them! Religion as a weapon rather than a way to save those in need. Some people were apparently not happy with my recovery. I don't feel sorry I let the air out of their hopes and went on living. I'm not talking about kids here. The young didn't care enough to do more than just pretend I don't exist. If only everyone could be that immature…

They have always, and still haven't stopped, trying to take my religion away from me. I won't go into the details, but I didn't get it from people, and people can't take it.

And then there was Amy. A year after I got out of the hospital (I was admitted in September 1992 at Cedars-Sinai) I took out that tape and letters (along with Suicidal Tendencies of course) and I listened to the tape again and read the letter again. I then decided that September would be Amy Appreciation Month. She was told by certain people not to get attached to me, though, because I have a severe illness. My illness would have had far less of an impact on my life if other people wanted to see me as a human being rather than some monster to be isolated and destroyed. The worse disease is not what is in me, but what was done *to me.*

When I got out of the hospital in 1992, I called Amy. The next day her mother called me, beginning by thanking me for being nice to Amy. Then she went into how Amy is too messed up to *deserve* friends (ADD). Her mother told me to *pretend* to be her friend, just to be nice. Obviously, I wasn't the only one people and their mothers are trying to isolate. That gave us something in common. (She also had roughly the same experience at a different Baptist school in Ridgecrest). Since Amy's mom isn't God (unless you ask her) she doesn't get to decide who I am friends with and it would go against my conscience to fake something. I would not become part of abuse by proxy, and certainly I wasn't going to treat people the way I had been treated since I was little. If one only listened to what society tries to claim is the way things are, (like that mothers love their children and would never do anything to hurt them or want them dead, even though there are countless cases in the news every day) one might not believe that someone's own mother would treat them like that. Like Crohn's disease, it can only be understood by someone who experiences it for themselves. To understand anything, it is first necessary to be willing to see things for what they actually are, not what they say something is *supposed to be.* Or what they want to *make it be.*

It isn't like I don't have social skills or am unaware of the usual society crap people use to meet people. It has more to do with the fact that I have no interest in tricking people into liking me. That would only attract the most shallow people anyway, with meaningless relationships that can never go anywhere. I only want what is real. I am only interested in deeper connection, so that I might be able to share the deeper things of life I have rarely been able to share to any degree. The counselor in 1990 was very confused by that. Through a psychological test he got the contradictory result that I consider friends important and also unimportant. The problem with a multiple choice question on a test is that limiting a response to only those select answer choices is the same as dictating the answer to the person taking the test. Those answer options were set up by someone who had a very limited view of reality and motivations. They were choosing answers for me, since I wasn't allowed to give my answer. I had no voice there. The questions were leading type questions that had little contact with reality. I consider friends important, but there are other matters which can't be compromised to obtain friends. Why is it so hard to get that across to someone claiming to be

Christian? They can make up whatever god they want but they can't force me to bow down to their idols. He asked me how many friends I have, and when I counted around ten, he expressed shock and acted like I was just making them up. He denied that it was even possible for someone like me to have friends! And this was the guy who was supposed to fix me. Fixing me also meant that I was supposed to hate myself since I was ordered to accept the hatred against me as right. When I wasn't breaking like he wanted, he also tried using the tactic of telling me that since his Baptist son wasn't hated at that school everything is fine and I am just making it up. One thing power freaks like to do is create a problem just so they can pretend to solve it. One psychological test I came across had the question "Would you rather be the center of attention or one of the crowd?" That is a leading question, and both of those choices are wrong. The reality is that the crowd is irrelevant. As an individual, people don't choose who I am, and they have no right to demand that I accept what they dictate. If the psychology world knew what self-esteem is they would see the contradiction in placing one's sense of value in the hands of those seeking to destroy.

Once, I when I was living in Riverside, I tried doing the shallow things others do to trick stupid people into liking them. It instantly worked. It was gross and dirty and I decided to never try that experiment again. I was shocked just how gullible people are. I was shocked by the double standards of those with such pretend ideals. I had hoped that at least that would be different outside of Ridgecrest. I saw people say one thing about values, but then I noticed who they would be tricked by. I could only feel disgust for them, having thrown away the values that they claimed as empty words people are taught to say but not mean, and they got their reward for stupidity. Too bad none of them wanted anything real. I would rather be alone than fake. A real friend would accept me for who I am. There were no friends in Riverside.

People I knew almost all fell prey to what I refer to as the "Who am I" trap. That trap consists of people taking cues from society when supposedly looking for who they are and looking everywhere except at themselves. Who you are is not going to be found outside of who you are. If the psychology world actually looked at the term "self-esteem" they would see the contradictions in what they preach. The term begins with the word "self". Isn't that where one should look to find themselves. It is stupid to place one's sense of personal worth in the hands of those seeking to destroy. Real validation comes from within. Any validation sought from external sources isn't real. Why, as the Bible asks, should people seek honor one from another, and yet seek not that honor which comes from God only? It is others who withhold personal worth from people, especially when someone is different. I refused to sell out, and they were unable to break me and convince me to hate myself.

I couldn't have survived without knowing myself. I would have given up and let myself die like I was told to do by my mother if I didn't have a personal sense of value. It is a nasty life, but at least it is mine.

Healing doesn't begin until the wounds stop.

4

There was a Saturday Night Live skit a while back about a medieval barber. Medieval medicine was pretty crazy stuff by today's standards. Barbers were the doctors, superstitions the science. In the skit, a woman was brought in very sick. The barber spoke about how advanced medical practice had become, how much more they know than they did before. The barber explained that previously they would consider the cause of that illness to be from witchcraft. But now they *know* that this condition is from an imbalance of bodily humors caused by a toad or small dwarf living in her stomach. The cure was to drain her blood…

Medicine does not necessarily proceed from myth to fact, but from one myth to a newer, more refined myth. As an example, I was still hearing in the 1990's that Crohn's disease was caused by my mother swallowing toothpaste while pregnant and it somehow damaged my intestines instead. I was told by doctors and nutritionists what to eat and what not to eat. No one ever got one thing right. I had to survive by observing what actually happens, which was often the exact opposite of what they said.

Most cases of Crohn's are less severe, and there is a large margin for people to do bad stuff and not necessarily notice. Even doctors have acted like this is just some inconvenience rather than a serious problem. One gets a more sobering view of it if they try to get life insurance with Crohn's disease. I've been through so many blood transfusions that I lost count in the early 1990s, but that doesn't stop doctors from denying that it is dangerous. Healthy people can and do make significant mistakes, but are healthy enough to get away with it. That which is OK for one person can kill another. I don't have a margin for error.

It was recommended that I talk with other people who have Crohn's for support. I quickly learned that I had little in common with other cases, or they just didn't understand. Every case is different, but doctors still treat it as if they are identical, and it is insulting to make the effort to see a doctor for this problem just to have them treat someone else's case but with me paying for it. It doesn't get me better.

Probiotics were recommended, especially acidophilus, and others. Those supposedly help people with Crohn's, and they do work for some people. I'm not one of those people. Most are very damaging to me, and one probiotic capsule is usually enough to put me in the hospital. Obviously, when something is wrong things don't work the same as they do for healthy people.

I was told to avoid fiber, with the myth being stated that it would make things worse by scraping the intestines away. How are the intestines supposed to work without fiber? When I moved to San Bernardino, I had little money, and I was eating cheap loaves of wheat bread that I could get for 30 cents at the time. It would last more than one day, and I couldn't afford much else. When I was reduced to that, I noticed that the more of the wheat bread I ate the more all symptoms were reduced. 100% whole wheat was even better, but I had to bake it myself to afford that. It is bleached flour which I have a slight sensitivity to. The fact is, the intestines can't function without fiber, and in my case wheat fiber was the only one with noticeable benefit. Other fibrous plants didn't help the Crohn's symptoms. Doctors and nutritionists kept telling me to stop eating wheat, even though it was helping me greatly. I wasn't stupid enough to follow their advice, and observable fact is more important than empty theory regardless of the source.

Doctors are just people, and they are just as vulnerable to myth and gimmicks and fads as anyone else. There is a war against wheat in society, but people lie about what wheat does.

Another is milk. Yes, there is a large number of people who don't tolerate milk, but I am not one of those. Doctors always tell me that milk will hurt me. One doctor told me to stop drinking milk because *he* is lactose intolerant! That is as stupid as the school teacher who told me that I like the color blue because I am a boy! That kind of behavior has always been a fast way onto my shit list. (My favorite color is gray, and no one has a right to take that away from me. Blue became a weapon for those who want to deny and destroy who I am as a human being to turn me into something I am not, besides the outright death threats I got from some of the blue pushers! I am not defined by a color, and I am person, not a pronoun. I can't be stuffed in a box, and certainly not someone else's box. No one has a right to dictate to me who I am, and I don't care what bogus Ethan they want to make up in their heads.) It would be nice for doctors to do their job and treat *my* case. That would take accepting proven observable facts and dropping blind suppositions. It would require *change* and *acceptance* of even the things that don't fit in with empty theory, no matter how pretty that theory is.

Another thing I observed was that a small amount of cocoa in something also had enough of an effect to notice. Whole wheat brownies had an edge over plain wheat bread. I noticed that it takes very little cocoa in something to aid digestion, which has confused doctors since there hasn't been any studies on that.

Another thing is heavily processed meats. Those may be bad in various ways, but when trying to survive there are other considerations. There is no future to get cancer in if I can't survive the present. Processed meats don't rot like other stuff does, although regular meats tend to not cause any problems if I am able to tolerate solid food at all, especially if I boil the hell out of it.

While in Riverside, I was doing quite bad. But one thing I did observe then was that even if I was having trouble with solid food and couldn't eat a hamburger, strangely I could eat a cheeseburger with no effects. That gave me a clue. I increased my milk intake as much as I could afford, and noticed that symptoms were also reduced by milk. The more the better. It wasn't hurting me in any way, even though the doctors all acted like somehow it would kill me. There is an anti-milk lobby, and they have been promoting the idea of milk being a poison. In their ads, they have used such tactics as claiming the effects of lactose intolerance as an absolute for everyone, including those who are not lactose intolerant! What they actually have a problem with is not the milk, but the conditions and treatment and exploitation of cows. I might have been willing to take their side if they weren't liars, but that would go against my conscience to go along with their lies, and that is aside from the fact that they want me to sacrifice my life to promote their agenda.

I don't recommend my diet for a normal person, and this diet is not my preference. It is just survival. Other people with Crohn's disease need to observe things for themselves and not just blindly obey some doctor who is only talking from theory rather than from personal experience. I won't say that my way of surviving is what would work for someone else's case. I don't care how things are *supposed* to work. Listening to the wrong advice can be deadly. Don't do something stupid just because someone has letters after their name.

I know the war on wheat has to do with harmful farming practices, but that lobby chose to lie instead of presenting their agenda honestly, so I can't support such groups since I can't support their methods of achieving their goals. You can't do what is right by doing what is wrong. I'm not stupid enough to condemn myself to death to appease some crowd of liars, regardless of their self-righteousness and sanctimonious egos. Why would they want me dead if they had such an interest in my health?

I also tried having a plant based diet. What I learned was that I lost the ability to absorb plant matter. It was like being NPO. I was losing a pound or more a day and getting too weak to function in just a few days. There was no combination of plant proteins that I could absorb. It has been that way since either my first surgery in 1989 or my second in 1992. Meat was generally unaffordable, but there was milk. Milk had the added benefit of being a liquid, and so I could survive on it when I couldn't have any solid food. It combined both food and water, which was important when I could only tolerate a low intake volume. It kept me alive, and I would not have been able to survive without TPN without milk. Vitamin supplements were used in combination with the milk, only I needed twice what a healthy person would need due to lower absorption. I was even told by doctors to not take those vitamins. Doctors also pushed Ensure, which I would have required at least a gallon of at that time (two gallons now) to match what I get from my stuff. (I did the calculations). The Ensure was worthless, and only contains a smaller number of essential things that someone could get from a bowl of cereal. It was also low on protein. The only reason I could think of why doctors were trying to get me to go into debt for Ensure was that they must hold stock in it. I could find no other reason.

Among the messed up advice I have been given by doctors, there was even the incident when a doctor recommended that I start smoking!

I would not be alive if I had gone against what I know. I grew up in a religion which teaches observing, and teaches going with what you know. It also teaches people that it is critical to know everything for yourself, and one can't rely on the word of others alone. We were taught that everything must be tested and proven. We also have a right to question anything and anyone and expect to get an honest answer, because that is how people learn. This is both a free will religion and a free thought religion, recognizing those rights in all people, not just our own, as stated in the articles of faith of the church. Without free thought one is not free to know or accept anything. Therefore there can be no faith in anything without free thought. We are also taught to look for truth wherever it is to be found, regardless of the source, because there is truth to be found everyone. If someone else knows something which will make us better people, we need them to share it with us. Religion is either personal or it doesn't exist. If it isn't personal then you don't really have it. If it isn't personal, it can be taken away by anyone. It was unfortunate witnessing the vast majority throw away such concepts.

There is a parable in the Bible which is given great importance, that is, for those who even care. It regards ten virgins waiting for a wedding. They waited long into the night, and their lamps went out. Five of them were prepared with extra oil for the lamps, and five weren't. The five not prepared asked the others for their oil. The five with oil couldn't give it, not because they were being selfish, but because of what the oil represents. All they had power to do was to tell the others to go and get oil, except now it was too late (the markets were closed). That oil is a type of knowledge, which one can't borrow from someone else. There is no such thing as borrowed faith. Talk is meaningless. Even if God came down and told you something, that does not mean that it is automatically true simply because you were told so. It is either true or not true, regardless of the source. Although, some sources have more credibility than others. Truth is self-existent. It doesn't need to be believed to be true. Lies only exist by being believed. Truth can be discovered, but neither created or destroyed, and will go on existing regardless of opinion. Look for truth within yourself. Either you have it within you or you don't. If you don't have it, you have to do what it takes to get it. It is in there, but it still has to be found to have it in a positive way. It can't be given, but it can be thrown away…Most people in that religion have tried to take it from me, spending their efforts to deny that I know this for myself, rather than getting it for themselves. There was an extreme of depravity that they were willing to go to. Murder was not beyond them, and was accepted by them as a legitimate means to achieve power. I wasn't part of the clique, and I'm glad I was never accepted so I didn't get blood on my hands from all the destroyed lives. If I hadn't mentioned it already, I ended up having to flee Ridgecrest under threat of death from them at the end of 1994, but it's not like people like that will ever let a victim escape.

If I hadn't learned for myself such concepts, things would have been very different. I was also taught about the value of all life, with the exception that people also tried to convince me that none of it applied to me. My mother opposed the religion in the home, and tried to deny the vast majority of it, even though she would put on a fake show of devotion every Sunday. My father was too weak to resist. He was not allowed to share things. Occasionally, he would open up quietly when we were outside away from my mother. I had to hold these things inside.

I was also taught that individuality is a divine gift, never to be taken away.

Healing is possible, in spite of the efforts of what has seemed to be all of society to prevent it. Real healing happens alone. But I have to wait for mine.

5

My own group was not the only one using religion as a weapon. I ended up at Loma Linda through insurance changes. It is a religious hospital with the hugest and most narcissistic self-promotion campaign I have seen from a hospital group. They are the self-proclaimed top of everything, in spite of what actual studies showed. Even though they have such a show of being Christian, once my religion was put on record, there was a very drastic change in demeanor toward me…

I had been seen at Kaiser for a time because an insurance change took me away from the effective care I was getting at Cedars-Sinai, and it has never made any difference which Kaiser facility I end up with. That was a disaster, and my health trouble went out of control. I had to quit my job to chase other insurance or I would be dead. Kaiser gave me the impression that they really didn't care if I lived or died, since that was the road they were taking me down. Ending up at Loma Linda was a way to try to get a referral back to Cedars-Sinai. I wouldn't have been able to function at all without the liquid diet (i.e. the evil milk) that I had been using, since I was going basically without treatment and lost tolerance for solid food. It bought me some time.

Enter Dr. Nick and Friends…

Loma Linda was a worse disaster than Kaiser. The religious façade made everything worse. I learned quickly that you can't ask people for help who view illness as a curse from God because I am supposedly so evil and therefore deserve it. Jesus spoke against victim blaming, including in health matters. If they would read the Bible for themselves, they would know that. Everything about their health care concepts were a reinforcement of their religion. They do many plant studies, or claim to study them, to try to show that their religious diet is the cure for everything. One can't look at how healthy those people are when they kick out anyone who gets sick as being a sinner. Their studies are frequently debunked and results unrepeatable outside of their group. All it does is prevent people from getting the help they need. Still, they proclaimed themselves to be the top of the nation, and more advanced than anyone else (actually I found them to be at least ten years behind other hospitals in both knowledge and technology, and that even included Kaiser).

Beside the incompetence, they had money problems. Their Christian pretensions didn't prevent them from engaging in such practices as moving extra equipment into my room (they said they just needed to clear space in another room and needed to put the equipment in my room just to get it out of the way) within minutes of an auditor checking my room and marking down ALL equipment present as in used. Not to mention the slight oxygen leak which for some reason could never be fixed (I was not on oxygen but the leak was still put on the bill). There is no such thing as a religion when money gets involved.

Loma Linda was a nightmare. I had a number of health problems by now, 2003. I had severe osteoporosis. I had kidney problems caused by cyclosporine treatment. I don't blame anyone for that. The cyclosporine undid all the damage that Kaiser did to me. It wasn't Loma Linda who helped me with that. It was at Cedars-Sinai, where I was able to get a referral to from Loma Linda to treat the Crohn's problem. As long as I was able to get to Cedars, the Crohn's problem was under enough control most of the time.

At Loma Linda, health care took very strange turns. I was referred to a nephrologist. Nice guy, very willing to help, but he had his own sleep issues. In my first visit, he started out by telling me that I needed a transplant. The next visit, no transplant necessary. The third visit, I need a transplant. Every visit alternated like that. He was helpful in giving me blood, for which I was grateful, which I run low on. The toad is still living in my stomach, and losing and replacing countless units of blood hasn't gotten rid of it…

There was even a battle of the nephrologists which occurred during a stay in the hospital. One nephrologist came in and wanted me on diuretics. Another doctor came into the room shortly after and said no diuretics. A third doctor came in after that, also saying to put me on diuretics. I mentioned what the previous doctor said about no diuretics, and that doctor dismissed it as nonsense. Five doctors got involves in the diuretics argument, which only discredits all of them. I got out of the hospital soon after that. I got a phone call from a doctor telling me that he had prescribed the diuretic and to take it immediately. I went to the pharmacy and picked it up, and by the time I got home I got another phone call telling me not to take it. It would be easier to get medical advice from a Magic 8 Ball, which is more credible than some doctors.

The most disturbing stuff at Loma Linda happened when I developed a Nocardia infection. That caused both pleural and pericardial effusions, which were very painful, and caused heart trouble and difficulty breathing unless I am upright. I went into the hospital, and got admitted. They could see nothing wrong, even though the bulging fluid was visible under the skin. It was also a coincidence that going in when I did caught one of the massive bleed-outs I go through every so often, since my Crohn's problem attacks major blood vessels in my intestines. I was given a few units of blood a day for a week, and then the bleeding slowed down enough that I only needed blood once a month or so after.

They kept checking my heart, and finding nothing unusual, so they were going to send me home. I kept telling them about the fluid, but they wouldn't listen. They would tell me "That's impossible." One doctor I showed the fluid to poked at my chest, said again that it is impossible that it could be a bulge of fluid, and insisted that I just don't have a sternum. My sternum shows up on radiographs just fine. Eventually, someone got the idea of doing a echocardiogram. The fluid showed up just fine in that, even though the technician doing it also told me it was impossible.

The nurses were bad enough, but the doctors I dealt with while in the hospital were dangerous. They were making mistakes every day which made me afraid to go to sleep. They refused to let me see lab test results, yet didn't seem to know how to read the results themselves. One example is when my potassium level was under 3 and they decided to give me kayexalate. I forgot to refuse until they told me the result which they pretended they had looked at, and then they were scrambling to keep my heart from ripping itself apart.

The We Know Everything attitude continued. Even after surgery for the infection, they went back to telling me that the fluid building back up in my chest was impossible, even though they had already seen it. I was in the hospital again, since I couldn't get competent treatment for the infection, and in desperation to get help from them, I had to go to the extreme of pulling out my hidden emergency razor blade I kept around, cut my chest open with it and showed them the fluid pouring out! That was how far I had to go to try to get help in a hospital that claims to be the best. Emergency razor blade are something hard to live without and you just can't think ahead of time what you will need one for.

But, those were Dr. Nick clones, and were doing this stuff out of incompetence rather than malice. That was to change with what happened next when they assigned me an infectious disease doctor.

Some studies have been more positive with female doctors. Those weren't the ones I ended up with. Most I met turned out to be flaming narcissists. They won't listen. Some were willing to say sympathetic sounding things about how sorry they are that I have health problems. I don't go to a doctor to be patronized. It would have been better to give me a solution rather than words. I'm not interested in theatrics. Pretending to care is an insult and doesn't mitigate failure. Also, just because media calls something "mansplaining" doesn't mean that women don't do it even more. The exception has been at Cedars-Sinai, which was different even in the narcissist realm. I can actually feel respected as a person at Cedars-Sinai, even with the female nurses and doctors. Other places have very bad hiring practices. I can't think of any pathological liars that I met at Cedars-Sinai.

The infectious disease doctor they put me with was even worse, combining both the incompetence with her narcissistic malice. I was treated with extreme contempt. Her incompetence resulted in many relapses over a year and a half. She would only do just enough to look like she was trying to help, but kept me from getting better, but that was only when she was even bothering to pretend. She also denied everything I said. That included about the fluid, which had been proven repeatedly to exist. She went beyond denying my pain to at one point even mocking my pain. Nothing she said was right and I had to continually correct her regarding what I was experiencing, and she was very hostile to me. I had to confront her about the failures of the treatments and being pulled off treatment before it was effective. She would start a treatment and then suddenly stop it before it could be effective. She asked me how many cases of Nocardia I've treated, even though I haven't seen her treat even one case (like mine.) I told her that I deal with my case, which she was supposed to be dealing with. She eventually went into a rage during one visit when she couldn't keep denying the facts of the fluid, and she dictated an order in front of me for my sternum to be removed! I saw that she was very dangerous and would rather have me die that face her failure. I had to get out of there fast. I even got a job with a company to change insurance again and get back to Cedars-Sinai. I saw an infectious disease doctor there who got the infection under control in two weeks and there have been no relapses since then. I didn't imagine that in the future I would meet even deadlier doctors than that. I had gone through a year and a half continual relapses because of her only pretending to treat the case but purposely preventing it from being cured by her denial of treatment tactics. She kept me sick with a very deadly problem that long and I was lucky to have lived.

I'm still upset about them leaving me on a ventilator that didn't work right after a surgery. They were supposed to have me on it for maybe two hours after. They didn't understand that it was malfunctioning and refused to take me off of it because they said I had the problem, not the machine they didn't know how to run. Somehow it is always *me* who has the problem and everything is just fine! I've heard that my whole life. I was on it for a couple days, in a never ending state of near suffocation, with unknown damage done. Eventually the surgeon came by and saw me on it and freaked out and ordered me removed from it. Of course, I could breathe just fine when they aren't stopping me!

Religion as a weapon. All this time dealing with fake Christian care, problems followed me to San Bernardino in the church there. The hatred was unpleasant. The women there were the worst, like in Ridgecrest. They had ties to the people in Ridgecrest, so they continued the abuse for the Ridgecrest people since I wasn't directly reachable by the Ridgecrest people. Mercenaries. I was being constantly reminded of how evil I must be because I was born with a severe illness. I was told constantly that if I had faith I would have been healed, therefore I must not have faith. Can't they see the miracles? It was only the women saying that to me, but it was all of them. So much for women having some sort of natural compassion. I know this group doesn't have it, therefore compassion must be a learned behavior, and these particular women missed some lessons somewhere. They all know about Saint Paul and his "thorn in the flesh" which he was not healed from. But that was OK for him, not me. For Saint Paul it was a sign of his faith, for me a sign that I am just a faithless devil and I deserve anything done to me. I have seen miracles just as impressive as those in the Scriptures. I can't share them though. It should have been enough for them to see my survival as a miracle, my overcoming difficulties as a witness of my faith. Rather than ascribing the power of God to why I was still around when I should have died a number of times, they even ascribed the power of the devil to me!

    Can a shadow exist when light shines upon it?
    There is rests unseen
    In plain sight defying recognition
    Shining forth in invisible brilliance
    Eclipsed in judgment by those who wish it weren't so.

I had to learn that there is help, but help usually comes when I am already falling off the cliff, even in the form of a tiny literal weed on a ledge that somehow had the supernatural power to hold me when it shouldn't have. Then suddenly I'm back on the road like it never happened, it makes no sense, but there I am. I have always known that I will be helped when the time comes. It doesn't have to make sense. I don't have to be able to explain a fact to know not to argue with the result. I only have to know help is there, even though I may never be released from my thorn in the flesh. I don't have to worry. My device keeps spinning, and people haven't found a way to pull the plug.

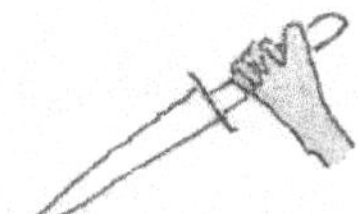

Inpatient Services

Expecting us to do our job ___________________________ $92600.00

Falsified tests___________________________ $31920.00

Treatments never administered___________________________ $5400.00

Unrepairable leaking oxygen meter___________________________ $6200.00

Unused equipment in another room___________________________ $15310.00

Common sense fee___________________________ NA

Patient asking questions___________________________ $21150.00

Malfunctioning equipment___________________________ $62000.00

Expired food___________________________ $590.00

Have a nice day, or don't, we really don't care.

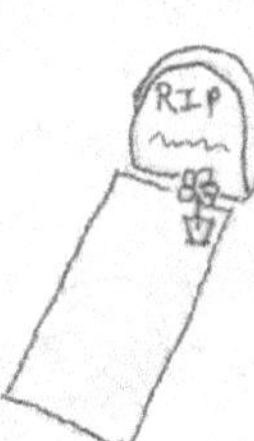

6

Why will I be bringing up the stuff in this chapter? Because the predators come when they smell blood, and with needing countless transfusions there was always plenty of fresh blood to smell. (Please donate as much Type O+ as possible – I need all I can get). Something as incapacitating as Crohn's disease makes one a target. Friends can be an important source of strength, but they have to be real friends or they don't count. Those called friends are also a target for those who don't want someone to be helped. There has to be safety, a place of refuge, for there to be healing of any sort. That is why they make such an effort to keep me from being safe anywhere. What happened can't be separated from the fact that I have Crohn's disease, for that is one of the weapons turned against me. I learned long ago that my only safe place is the one I carry inside me. Peace is wherever I can find it. Safety is where there are no people, since people are the danger. If it wasn't for what people have done to me I would probably have had a vastly different outcome in treatment of the disease. That even created a vicious spiral, with bad treatment creating a condition for me that people then were able to use a proof of me being evil and punished by God and even more deserving of everything they did and were doing to me. These experiences can't be separated from the disease. They happened because of it.

A disease is not just physical, it is also social, emotional and spiritual. All things are connected and it is all of those things which make the experience what it is. Healing the physical may be great, but it is not the only damage done by a physical problem. When one part of it is being treated the other parts carry on. Some people have support systems, others don't. It is necessary to find ways of coping with all of them. Serious problems can take away anything, except who we are, which can only be lost by throwing it away by choice. Things just slip out of grasp in the bad times. "Friendships" evaporate when someone needs help. Job from the Bible saw that, when those who had previously acted as friends came not to comfort him but to rip him apart for having a problem. Victim blaming. It makes weak people feel better and more powerful when they can make someone else worse than they see themselves. Attacking the vulnerable makes the truly weak feel less vulnerable, like something could never happen to them because of how superior they want to pretend they are. That is why so many people blame rape victims. It is easier for them to do that so they can go on pretending that something could never happen to them rather than face their fear. They can tell themselves that they are safe because somehow the victim deserved it and they don't. Jesus talked about victim blaming. The physical problem is not malicious, it is just a problem that happens, a circumstance. People are another matter. Deliberate harm comes from people, both direct harm, and the harm caused by deliberately interfering with help in order to keep a problem going. There is no difference. The end result is the same.

If all I had was the physical, there would be no way to continue. There is more to life than grasping for what isn't mine to have. There is more to experience than Crohn's Disease, although it had great influence on all of those experiences, both in shaping them and in limiting them. There were experiences that get me through all of the things which have happened. I didn't forget. I didn't throw those away. I hold them sacred.

In a very dark moment of my life, 1993, I had gone through the terror people tried to inflict on me, and surviving certain attempts had a profound effect and opened my mind to things beyond. My eyes were opened while looking at a tree, and I could see it's very life. I saw life after not giving up on my own in the face of unpleasant odds. One night, thinking of those attempts and looking again at the tree, I found myself outside at midnight contemplating survival, and I found myself listening to birds sing. I thought of the life of the tree and how my eyes were opened so I could see it. I thought of the manner in which I had been prevented from being murdered. I still step outside at midnight now and then to listen to the birds and re-ground myself in what I was shown then, which was more than just the tree experience.

In 1996 I was contemplating the experience and wrote:

When the shadows stretch across the land
Do your heart and mind turn black?
Or do your ears and spirit fill with all that the daylight hours lack?
Have you let the chilly seasons drag you down into despair?
Now throw down your chains of sorrow as the songbird's music fills the air.
Has stress filled your mind with blindness
Or can you hear the notes so sweet?
Lay aside your daily worries and enjoy your midnight treat.
Warmth and light for those who look
Hymns of comfort for those who hear
You're never alone in the darkest hours
The Comforter is always near.

I was protected, yet in a way on my own in the usual sense. Almost all people who had been friends at some time turned on me, and I'm happy to let them go. Those friendships were one sided anyway, and I couldn't keep that up with people who clearly didn't want anything to do with me. I have to just keep going on my path without them since they wouldn't walk this road with me. I have to stay true to my path. It is all I have.

It would be wonderful to find out I was adopted, but I know I wasn't. Narcissists attack anyone who has a weakness, and in this family I was the "scapegoat child" who had to be hated no matter what. No success ever meant anything. My drugged up wife-beating brother was the "golden child" who could never do wrong. My brother is also as bad of a narcissist as my mother, from having learned it from her. Of course, growing up, I was hated by him for having an illness, and I had to be on my toes at all times. It is what can be called abuse by proxy. He was told to hurt me, and he was allowed to do anything he wanted to me without consequence. The object of that tactic is that he would be blamed, and he deserves it, but that my mother would not take any blame even though she was the one provoking him and I knew it. She would pretend to try to comfort me, but she would only betray me. I always had to be ready to flee home forever growing up, with an escape plan in place from a young age. I did have to run to save myself at one point but I was talked into coming back. I learned to sense people approach me in my sleep, and I was always ready to strike, which occurred. That instinct never left me. It can't leave me. Danger never left, even to this day.

Since support is so important in dealing with a major illness, isolation was one of the tactics used to prevent me from having support. They all abandon me. My mother would insinuate herself into any friendship to gain influence. I grew up watching her isolate others. She would call someone who is a "friend" and talk about that person's friend. She would tell them of the sinister convoluted plots supposedly taking place and how that other friend is just using that person. Having warned them of the dangerous person that they knew for many years and had no idea what a monster they supposedly are, my mom would then call up the horrible monster she just warned about and give them the same speech about the first person. The people would then break their friendship, isolating them, leaving my mom in control of them. She would throw in how only she is smart enough to see what is really going on. She wouldn't stand any competition, such as people having a personal life she isn't in control of.

She also had a spy network, known in the psychology world as "flying monkeys" in reference to the Wizard of Oz. Those are people who are willing to go along with the abuse by proxy, to spy on the victim, and also to engage in destructive behavior, striking when the opportunity comes. She would say that I was seen at a place and they reported it to her. I was supposed to think that she knows everything. The point of the tactic was not that she does know anything, but to get me to break down and give her the information she is too stupid to just observe directly. I can recognize information mining and didn't fall for it. I mapped out her spy network. I can't ever respect those people who would do that to someone simply because they were told to.

Some people took a more professional approach to the terror, even hiring people to follow me in Ridgecrest. One was a ridiculous investigator who would follow me when I would be out walking. He was a joke. How was I not supposed to notice someone slowing down while driving near me and talking into a recorder while staring at me? I pretended not to notice, but he was there all over the place. With someone like him around, I knew anyone who meant harm wouldn't do anything to me right then since he could be spotted so easily. I can't prove who hired that clown, but I can guess. The members of the church also hired a real spook to terrorize me, which was directly admitted by them...

Health care is important, so that was under attack also. My mother wanted me dead at least for most of my life. She hated me and said so, and I was more valuable to her dead than alive because of the sympathy she could get. She tried to convince me to give up insurance so I wouldn't be able to get care. She also told me repeatedly to give up and let myself die, whispering it to me when other people wouldn't hear.

Another person even told me outright that he was going to use my illness to kill me. Oops, I mentioned one of those others who contacted me in the hospital in 1992 that I wasn't supposed to bring up.

It wasn't just me she was doing this stuff too. There is a trail of bodies she has left behind. All it takes is her pretending to care about a sick person and then when she has that person's trust she tells them that she doesn't like their doctor and they should stop getting the help keeping them alive. It worked on countless victims, complete with her even laughing about it on one occasion I remember. My son has Crohn's Disease also, and she went as far as to get a chiropractor to write that the gastroenterologist is all wrong about it and the treatment should be stopped. She also kept contact with my doctors...

And then there was Amy. Crohn's disease is what brought us together in 1992. It was a platonic friendship for a long time until other events occurred. We didn't rush into anything. Because I was sick, other girls at church were warned not to get close to me. A leader at the church even told me that it would be wrong for me to be in a relationship because I'm sick. Amy was warned too, but jumped in anyway.

When we got married against the opposition, there was an incident a few weeks later while visiting her family in Ridgecrest. Her mother, who ironically just happens to have the name Karen, was an even more extreme narcissist than mine. Amy also grew up as the scapegoat child. In that visit, her mother came up to me and told me that Amy doesn't take care of me like she does. (The mother actually did nothing to care for me and had no interest in any of my needs, and even though I may be in bad shape I take care of my own needs and I am not interested in people doing stuff for me, especially meaningless society show crap. To have a real marriage one has to give up false social constructs, and gender role trash has no place in a real relationship, and anything other than a real relationship is worse than meaningless. I didn't get married for "help" with anything and that is not my interest. Marriage has to do with two equal partners, and no one can become one if there is any degree of subordination. I only want what is real, and so I only want a real marriage, not "playing house" which any three-year-old can do with no meaning). The first part of the Cinderella story may have been about Amy's life growing up. Her mom then ordered me to punish Amy. She can't tell me to do that. I was very disgusted that she would want someone to hurt her daughter, but that wasn't the first sign of the abuse her family all heaped on her all her life. I'm not a mercenary and I'm not going to engage in the abuse by proxy everyone else she knew is willing to do. Her mother then began screaming at me to punish her NOW. I wouldn't do it. One classic sign of narcissists is the cartoonishly exaggerated gender role stereotypes that have no place in the modern world. Ever after that incident, her mom kept telling her to get ready to leave me because I was going to drop dead any moment and she needed to get away before that happened so she wouldn't be hurt by my death. Crohn's disease was combined with the usual gaslighting as an extra weapon, now to try to break up our marriage for my refusal to do something unconscionable. Her whole family got involved in that. I wasn't playing the game right, and they all wanted me dead for it. Before we were married, she had been told by her family that she is a bad daughter/bad sister. Then when we were married she was told by them that she is a bad wife. They then threw in that we shouldn't have children because she would be a bad mother, and that was all even said before we were married too. I wasn't as easy of a target as they hoped.

There was of course great hostility from the members of that church who wanted me dead. They hated Amy too, as they had all been told to by her mother. One might think that they would have been glad to be rid of people they have such intense hatred toward, but that isn't how predators operate. Narcissists destroy anything they can't have. They engage in abuse by proxy as I call it when they can't reach someone directly themselves. They don't care so much about who does the dirty work, as long as they can see the victim suffer. They like it even more when they have someone set up to take the blame for them. When we were married and living in Highland, all the hatred followed us there with just as much directed toward Amy.

None of this ever ended, and the campaign of terror goes on today.

Amy's family also exploited her weaknesses to break her down. She disobeyed a command from them and we had a son. While I was in Loma Linda trying to survive their treatment on top of the Nocardia infection, Amy's mom decided to strike while Amy was going through an anxiety attack. She came down to San Bernardino while I was sick and in a weakened state, and convinced Amy that she can't handle being a mother and ordered Amy to give up. Amy wasn't into listening to me, since she had been ordered to obey her mother without question no matter how self-destructive the order. She had been taught that it would be a sin to stand up to such evil and do what is right, even though Jesus taught people to do what is right, and even disobey family rather than be destroyed by them. That isn't the popular view of Jesus, but it is in the Bible. Now illness was destroying our family, but only because of people, not the disease itself. Amy's family wanted Quinn to be dead too. They didn't want him to even be born. They were intent on making him disappear…

One moment when I got out of the hospital, and Amy's mom was still around breaking Amy down with awful abuse, to the point of Amy curled up in a ball in the corner from the awful things her mom was yelling at her, I found that her mom had turned on the dryer and opened the back door. The house was filling with fumes. She had set Quinn right at the door two feet from the dryer vent. I ran over and got him and closed the door so he wouldn't die. Amy's mom ran over screaming at me that the door needs to be open (for fresh air she said even though it was filling the house with fumes which weren't in the house before she opened the door) and said that she put Quinn there and that was where he needed to be. She had tried to kill our son. I stood up to her and she ran off. Paper tiger, as they say. There was constant passive-aggressive tactics used, and she got Amy to tell me how mean I am to her mom, and how ungrateful I am for all the help. After saving our son's life from a murderer. Of course, we didn't have so many problems before her mom came, and Amy was in a much better mental state before her mom came to break her down. The predator had smelled blood, and not just mine.

Also, the constant gaslighting from all her family went in many directions to try to break us up. One thing was convincing Amy that since I was essentially already dead that she can't rely on me and can only rely on her mother. That made cooperation within our relationship difficult to impossible. We started out with a very stressful first year, with me having two bowel surgeries in the first half of it. One was a by-pass attempting to open up the narrowing, but it failed and I had to have it resected. Amy was there, but I was both married and going through these things completely alone at the same time thanks to the narcissists who were cheering for my death so they could get their slave back.

They had other means to dispose of Quinn. There was still my mother they could use, who was willing and capable of doing anything to anyone with no remorse and with little incentive needed.

Amy's mom convinced my mom that she should take Quinn as her own son. Not listening to me made this a very dangerous situation, and Amy's mom gave her the orders to go along with it and leave me and move in with my mom in Ridgecrest where she wouldn't have my support to resist.

Attempts were made to break me, making things as difficult as possible. The abuse Amy went through back in Ridgecrest was driving her to be suicidal. There is always a high suicide rate around narcissists, but it is really murder, since that is the goal of the abuse. My mother wanted to take Quinn as her own son, which she had also tried to do with other children. She did what she could to make him as entitled and narcissistic as possible, and especially worked to try to make him hate me and Amy as much as possible. She taught him to treat people quite awful, which meant he was not able to make real friends. His only "friends" were kids who were bribed into pretending to be his friends. That whole pretending to be someone's friend, just to seem nice, sounds familiar. She was isolating him and setting him up to fail at everything. She would encourage anger and violent behavior. If he hit someone, she would tell him that it wasn't his fault, it was their fault for getting in the way of his fist. That was literally said.

Quinn also has ADD like Amy, but since Quinn was being told he was perfect and being told that Amy was bad, she made up stuff about him being autistic so he wouldn't think he had something in common with Amy. I overheard my mother teaching him to act autistic because of all that they could get from the county programs if he acts that way. It was coached. He wasn't autistic before then and he stopped those behaviors when they were finally able to escape back to San Bernardino.

Among other parenting techniques she also took silverware away from him and from then on forced him to eat everything with his hands. There were too many things like that to even discuss in this book.

And then there were the phobias. Those were coached also. He didn't have those fears when living in San Bernardino. My mother would tell him that he was going to freak out over this and that, and he followed her cues. He had a trained anxiety after that, which took many years away from her to get over, yet began improving immediately when he was finally away from her. He had been a very happy child before that move to Ridgecrest. All this stuff was to isolate him so that my mother would be the only one he could trust, and my mother would be the only one he could be around, with all the dislike of him being spread around, and afraid to leave the house and see that there is a whole world outside of my mother. And he was also becoming exactly like my brother in every way.

Just to make sure that he didn't learn anything empowering, she taught him to fake a religion and treat it as a meaningless game to put on display but never learn anything about. It was this religion that gave me so much ability to resist her growing up, and not break. She didn't want that happening again.

He developed Crohn's disease also. I was trying to get him help for that, but my mother was trying to prevent help. I was even able to get Amy to take him to Cedars-Sinai for evaluation. That was deliberately sabotaged by my mother, who kept sneaking Quinn ibuprofen in significant amounts, which caused intestinal bleeding. She knew what the effect would be, since she remembered the warnings about ibuprofen from when I was growing up. The doctor, of course, was told about the ibuprofen by her, which, even though there were pictures from the endoscopy showing the bleeding sores all over and inflammation, they were dismissed as ibuprofen damage. So he was prevented from getting help and was kept sick by my mother.

Other means were also used to prevent treatment for Quinn. My mother took him to various doctors, anyone who would say what she wanted them to say. Any doctor who saw the truth was automatically a bad doctor and she wouldn't allow Quinn to see them. One gastroenterologist warned her directly about the damage she was doing to Quinn, but saying that to a malignant narcissist simply made her do it even more against medical advice. Much damage was done. She even got a chiropractor to read a blood test and review medication and write saying that the gastroenterologist is all wrong and Quinn must be taken off of medication. Narcissists do things like that so they have someone they can point the finger at when they are caught, claiming to be following their advice. She can't claim ignorance since she was going against everything she knew with my case. Quinn would have been dead very early if they hadn't eventually got out of there. She was also hiding ingredients in his food that were known allergies proven by testing. She was purposely keeping him sick.

Where was Amy in all of this? She was too broken to stand up for either herself or Quinn. Every time she saw what was going on and would be about to leave, her mother would break her back down and order her to stay, and repeatedly ordered her to give up Quinn. My parents even went so far as to take Amy to a lawyer and tried to force her to sign away her parental rights, but she refused.

I would visit when I could. There were attempts to make that as hard as possible, and to make sure Quinn would not be available when I could get there.

Amy's mother would call my mother and give her instructions on the abuse she wanted her to give Amy. Things would get especially bad after Amy's mother would call. Amy's family praised and supported everything that my mother was doing, since it was the same abuse they had all always participated in and what they all wanted done to her. They would do it directly like they used to if they hadn't moved to Colorado and Nevada.

It was a friend of ours who was finally able to get through to Amy and get her to see that what was happening was wrong. Amy was then able to think about leaving without as much of a guilt trip. Amy hadn't listened to my warnings. She had been trained to ignore anything I say. Even when the abuse would be severe enough that she would decide that leaving was best, they would break her down again and the next day Amy would tell me how righteous my mother is and how "ungrateful" I am. They (both our mothers and the rest of Amy's family) were able to make Amy feel that she was being evil by thinking of leaving, and she had been trained to believe she has to obey every command from her mother, and even her younger sisters, without question.

An email was forwarded to us. In this email (which we still have) there was a plot laid out to get Amy and Quinn to visit Colorado, then they were going to have my mother come and kidnap Quinn while they hold Amy there. I was never supposed to see either Amy or Quinn again. They also discussed trying to make me lose my house, since Amy's mother warned, as long as we have this house in San Bernardino Amy could legally take Quinn and move back. In a later message my mother gave me, she also mentioned that if she could go back she would have made us lose the house. That wasn't implied. It was stated directly.

A friend stepped in and gave Amy the support she needed to finally break out of there and get back to San Bernardino. Quinn immediately began improving in health once back. It made a huge difference for him to not be poisoned (literally poisoned.)

7

A friend enters the picture.

In 2013, I was in between insurances a couple times. Unfortunately, I ended up back with Kaiser, and didn't have an option. Things fell apart with my health again. There was a long interruption in my treatment, and it took a while to get back on Thalidomide. (My sleep dropped to around 2-3 hours a night, which didn't help.) My mother, of course, had been trying to convince me to give up my work and insurance so I wouldn't be able to survive, as well as trying to get me to give up my house so I wouldn't have a place to live.

It didn't look like I had much chance of surviving long, and with the family situation, it was getting too hard to survive. Support came from a friend from a long time ago. I was able to keep going, though in very bad and unstable shape.

Through some random incident searching the internet, the friend came across articles on narcissism, and showed them to Amy. Every tactic was an exact match. Amy was able to see these behaviors in my mother, but through her programming her mother and the rest of her family (with the exception of her father who she was allowed to hate) could never be seen as doing anything wrong, even though they were doing the same stuff.

Through bogus sob stories my mother was telling people at the church, she was able to grift what appeared to be thousands of dollars from people. Then, even while claiming how poor she is, she paid cash for another property in another town. It is hard to feel sorry for those people. They were all willing to go along with the abuse, and were willing to acknowledge my mother as Quinn's mother like she told them too, even with Amy right there. They were willing to treat Amy as not being Quinn's mother, and would ignore her completely and only interact with my mother in matters related to our son. I can't feel sorry for those people. They went against what they know to be true and were willing to support the abuse. They didn't do what they did in ignorance.

They were also willing to spy on us for my mother. We were harassed by former acquaintances in Ridgecrest who were ordered to contact Amy to make her feel wrong for leaving.

The joke was on them. Narcissists don't support their followers. They are only there to be used. In one case, Amy was a friend of one woman in Ridgecrest who had emphysema. Amy was assigned by the church to help her. My mother claimed to be the only on helping and denied that it was Amy helping. There was then a shuffle of people at the church and two women were assigned to help. My mother contacted them and ordered them to not help. She eliminated the competition. Then my mother convinced to sick woman to give up her car, so she was then completely dependent on my mother to get to doctor appointments. Then, like the usual predatory pattern of my mother, she told her she wouldn't take her to see that doctor anymore because my mother didn't like that doctor. The real reason was because that doctor was actually helping, and my mother enjoys watching people die. We tried to help that sick woman. We explained what was happening and what was going to happen if she didn't break away from my mother. Amy kept in contact with her after leaving Ridgecrest. That woman pretended to go along with what we were warning her about. The reality was that she was talking to Amy to get Amy to give her information to feed to my mother. Her betrayal of us forced us to break contact with her for our protection. She didn't do anything in ignorance. It turned out that she was a narcissist also, and narcissists always back each other up against a victim, and they don't care what damage they do to themselves as long as they get their power trip.

A friend from long ago helped Amy get out of Ridgecrest. That friend also tried to help that sick woman, but my mother got her to hate that friend. More competition eliminated.

Back in San Bernardino, Amy was constantly harassed by people trying to break her down. My mother used her connections in the church in San Bernardino to enlist the people around us in the campaign of terror she and Amy's family had planned. They tried to convince Amy to not have anything to do with that friend from long ago, who was the only friend Amy had now. They were all very angry that Amy escaped. They, including Amy's family, ordered

Amy to give Quinn to my mother. That behavior never ended and is still going. The women's president at the church was also enlisted to break Amy down, calling her just a few days after Amy moved back, and she told Amy that she can't make it as a mother, telling her to give up. She used identical words that Amy's family used. They all tried to convince Amy that I am very evil, and told her that she had to escape for her life. Even though they all (including Amy's siblings) said that they were going to "fix" Amy by getting her to Colorado, locking her in a place, and not allow her to do anything unless they told her to (they wanted her to be the slave for them like before), and that she would never see me or Quinn again, they said that I was the one trying to isolate her and control her. They claimed that the old friend was trying to break us up, even though they were the ones trying to break us up since we got married at the end of 1996. If I was trying to isolate Amy, obviously it would have happened immediately, like what my brother would do to anyone he could get to move in with him. If it was my sinister plot to isolate her, how come she has always been able to go visit her family any time and talk freely to them any time? They know all that, but that is how gaslighting works. They wanted her to be afraid, afraid enough to break.

They spread around the church in San Bernardino that I was having affairs, and also that our son isn't actually our son and that we kidnapped him. We have their kidnapping plot in writing in the email forwarded to us, and they even attempted to carry it out in 2016. There were two other leaders in the church contacted and told to make us give up our son. They refused to do such a thing.

One example of where being sick comes into all this is in 2017 I was back in the hospital. Kidneys were failing along with other problems. I got to the point of hallucinating. At the time there was a hurricane in the Gulf States, and people had been getting their flooded houses taken over by alligators. So I was seeing alligator everywhere, with my hospital room full of cute, cuddly alligators that wanted belly rubs. I knew that it wasn't real, and I was aware that being incapacitated in a room of alligators would not go well. I liked the hallucination, with all the beautiful lizards, but I only want what is real, and those weren't real, as comforting as they were at the time. Kidneys weren't the only problem, with a doctor even saying to me that he had never seen numbers so bad in someone still alive. Others seemed to not understand why I didn't seem to care. I mentioned to them that I've been worse. They said, but I was supposed to be dead. Maybe, but I didn't have a near death experience this time, so I've been worse. Some still had a hard time understanding how I could be so nonchalant about it. If I could have bullets flying inches from my head without panicking (different asshole than the one who owes me a windshield) then I'm not going to panic just because my numbers are wrong. I have always held onto hope of life no matter what people have done to try to take that away from me, but I had been denied from a long time ago the *expectation* of life. Ironically, real alligators would have ended things for me quicker and far more mercifully than some of the doctors I have had, some I've mentioned and some I haven't mentioned yet.

Amy's mother found out and decided to strike. She was very excited that I was "finally going to die". She was able to get Amy to break and Amy was unable to resist. She came to San Bernardino under the pretense of trying to help. She began throwing things away that we needed, and in general was just trashing our life any way she could (throwing out appliances, which included literally throwing things to break them). Her behavior was so bad that Quinn had to stand up for himself around her abuse, and Amy's mother pulled a knife on Quinn, which Quinn was able to stop her from using with a struggle ensuing. As already noted, that wasn't the first time she tried to kill him, and like typical narcissists still demand that he like them after all they have done to him (not just Amy's mom). That is the danger of having an illness that people are waiting to exploit. It is when I'm down that they strike. It is dangerous to let anyone know when I'm sick. Support from people is out of the question for us, but God always gets us through.

Amy tried asking the church for help while I was in the hospital. She asked the woman whose job it was to coordinate assistance, but Amy was told "No one would want to help *you*!" That, coming from self-proclaimed saints!

At one point, I lost a significant amount of blood in a few hours (20%). It stopped on its own, but it was related to the stress of the campaign of terror against us. That was aggravating the Crohn's problem. They had tricked Amy into going to Colorado, and the script was played out just like in the email two years before. Amy's father was able to get Amy to see through at least some of the gaslighting, and Amy was able to get out of there. During that trip, my mother had shown up to take Quinn, like they had planned. Amy caught her trying to poison him before they got out of there. Amy's family tried to claim that I am faking Crohn's in order to manipulate her.

I had eventually gotten away from Kaiser again, by changing companies again. I got back to Cedars-Sinai where they were able to stabilize me again. After a couple years though, I went through an insurance change and ended up back at Kaiser. Things fell apart much worse this time, although it took a little longer before I was back in an active flare-up, not that I can say I have ever truly been in remission, no matter how quiet it may seem at the times I get adequate treatment. My health falls apart every time I am with Kaiser.

Eventually, our friend from long ago turned on us too. That person also used a time I was in the hospital for a surgery. That person got information from Amy about my condition and then gave that information to multiple people who want to kill me, including one from a long time ago who had said he would come kill me at some time, the same person who had also said he would kill me through my disease long ago. She also told my mother about my condition so they could use the time of my weakened state to destroy us. We can never have anything to do with that person again. This wasn't the first time she spied on me and betrayed me to people planning to kill me. We had given her another chance, but she hadn't changed. That friend tried to get me to turn on Amy, telling me that Amy is really a narcissist and is faking ADD to manipulate me. That was laughable.

Among the things done to us to try to break us, Amy's family repeatedly called CPS. Each time the investigation showed none of the accusations to be true, such as the accusation that we don't have food and so Quinn has to wander the city begging for food. It was easy to show the investigator all our food that we have. There were many other bogus accusations.

Amy's family also exploited my weakness from surgery in 2020 by calling Adult Protective Services. Amy's sister sent me a card telling me how much they love me and want me to get better. That was an insult that she would think I would be tricked by that from someone who wants be dead and was literally cheering for my death. That trick was timed with the call to Adult Protective Services to make it appear that they were only doing that because of how much they care about me. Among the false accusations, one was that I was losing weight and getting dangerously weak, not from the surgery, but because Amy refused to feed me! The investigator found the accusation false, of course. (Even though the investigator had been told how crippled I supposedly was, supposedly unable to move or leave the bed, I was the one who answered the door, standing and walking around just fine without help!)

That is the danger of having a weakness in a predatory society. There are things which would never have happened if I didn't have bad health.

Among other things, they managed to get our utilities cut off. They also got someone to sabotage my truck to cause an accident, which goes along with them wanting me dead. That was timed on Quinn's birthday. A letter of no contact had been sent to my mother right before that because of her constant harassment, and we threatened to get an attorney involved if she didn't stop. It could have been anyone, especially people at the church in San Bernardino who would be willing to commit murder. I know of another case of one member of the church in Ridgecrest attempting to run someone down with his car. Guess who was considered the innocent one accepted by the members of the church, and which one had to flee for their life.

Real friends are defined by safety. They are not a threat. When dealing with as serious a problem as this, there is no margin for toxic people.

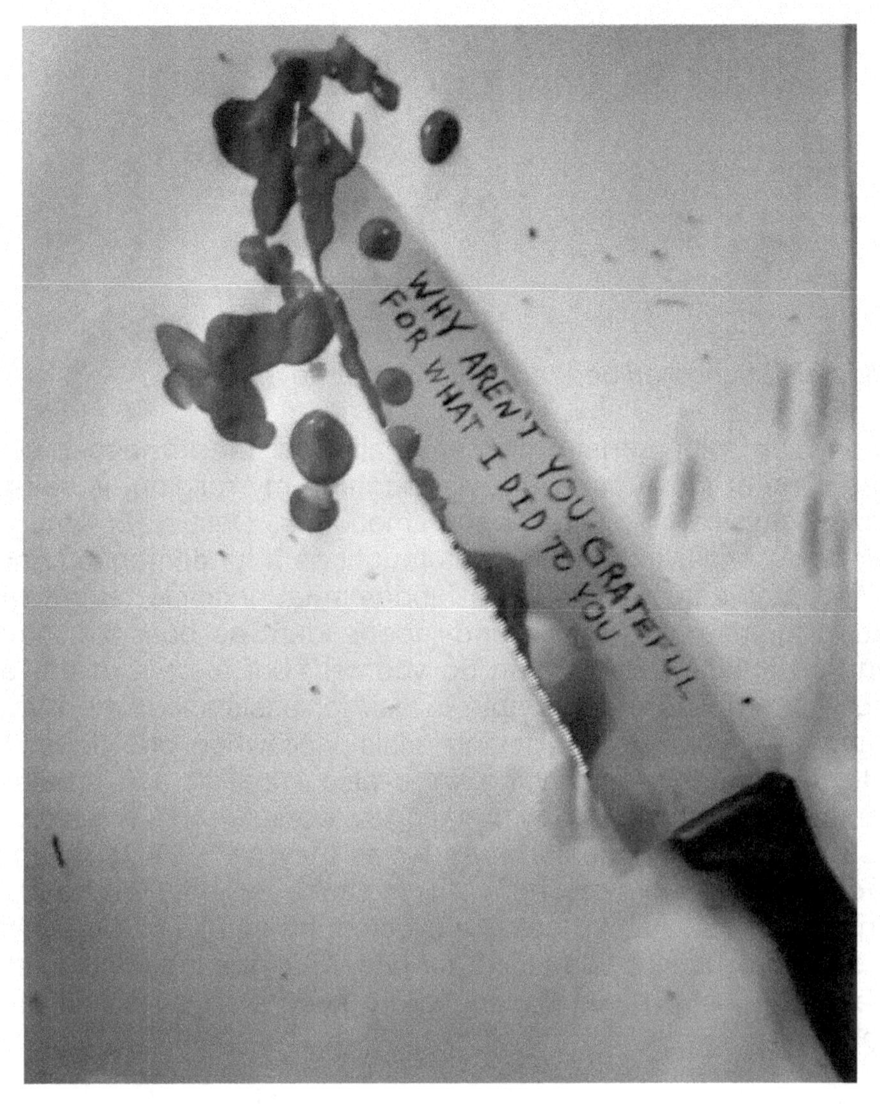

WHY AREN'T YOU GRATEFUL
FOR WHAT I DID TO YOU

8

Things lost, things gained, and things that never were.

Growing up with certain concepts allowed me to avoid certain fatal mistakes. One of those concepts, as taught in my religion, is self-reliance at all levels, physical, spiritual and emotional. Deliberate and *avoidable* dependency is enslaving. Freedom is taught as a fundamental principle to be maintained. Self-determination is a fundamental principle taught with it. One must keep themselves as free and independent as possible, never having someone do things that you can do yourself, but always at the same time knowing your limits and being able to ask for assistance when you can't do something on your own. Not getting assistance when one doesn't have the power to do something on their own is also crippling and creates a worse dependency than otherwise by creating a worse problem which had been avoidable. But one still should go as far as they can. Sitting down will never teach you to walk, and stopping will only cause atrophy. One early leader of my religion said that when there is a problem he can save himself faster than he can call a neighbor to come do it for him. That doesn't apply to all cases all the time, but is just a general guideline to keep as a goal. Not all goals are achievable.

Something I was taught also, but which other people of the religion missed, was a manner of studying. I was warned to set aside what people told me something means, and look at it fresh so that my interpretations would be based on what things actually say rather than distortions from what people want something to say.

Being sick taught me to be hated. It is just a simple fact in this society. What people call Darwinism and Social Darwinism is the rule of the day, and the excuse to treat anyone with a problem as an outsider, treat the sick person as the disease, to be eradicated not cured. A problem is viewed as a weakness, but God said that the weak will be made strong. A concept in my religion is the necessity of facing opposition. It is a grand teacher, as one works to overcome weakness. There is greater strength from facing opposition, because one is aware. The "strong" tend to be those who simply failed to recognize their weaknesses because they were never tried by opposition. How do they know they are strong? They are left only to prove their superiority by tearing down others. My disease didn't weaken me as much as people seem to want me weakened. Once again, it is the disease that has always surrounded me which is worse than the disease inside. Why do they WANT me to be weak? In one ridiculous incident, one narcissist spent hours demanding that I expose my weakness. He told me that friends help people with their weaknesses, therefore I am not being a friend unless I expose my weakness to him. He was a very dangerous person who later tried to get someone to kill me for him. I knew the way of the lizard. There is some real power there, as I will discuss below. Society makes people weak, which is required by the predatory nature of society.

In a Dr. Seuss story of the Sneetches, these creatures had a society where there was a group trying to form an exclusive clique. Someone came along peddling star imprints that could be placed on their bellies, thereby distinguishing the "special" ones from the others. They went back and forth with all the Sneetches adding or removing the stars. In the end, none were any more special or inferior than the other, except maybe in their own individual heads. It is the same in aristocratic groups of humans, with their hierarchies and cliques. There is the clique of the "normal", the supposedly *real* humans, just like the Sneetch clique claimed to be the *real* Sneetches.

There were other concepts I grew up with (taught from the church and certainly not at home.) One was the warning long ago that one can't blindly trust what someone else says is true. Everything must be verified. It was said that the wolves were already among the flock, wearing sheep's clothing because of the positions they hold within the church. One must know things for themselves or they don't know it at all. It is reality that matters, not words. Therefore it is reality and actual cause and effect relationships that have to be observed to be able to adjust to changing conditions in a serious illness. The myths floating around the medical world are a good example. Also the fact that one thing may be true in one case but not in another case.

A principle I learned, with the future always unpredictable, even within the same day, is to get as strong as possible in the good moments so that I would be as strong as I *have* to be in the bad times. That makes recovery possible, even when given the "failure to thrive" designation, which is considered to be hopeless. I've been written off as dead plenty of times, but most of those times were by people who want me dead.

How could I recover to any degree from the bad times unless I had practice fighting my way through these problems? How would I have developed the strength to keep going if I had given up like I had been ordered to by certain people? Without the opposition I faced since I was 7, I might not have been able to resist what people were doing to me and do what is right. With death as a near companion (no exaggeration), I had to have my priorities straight at a young age. Facing death many times made life far less frightening than people tried to make it for me. Death threats don't have the same impact…

There are different kinds of strength. If I couldn't develop my body at some time, then I would develop my mind, through meditation, learning and other stuff. That allowed me to face things people were trying to do to me without breaking. I survived some bad stuff, both natural causes from the disease and the stuff people were trying to do to me to make it worse. Does that make me the weak one, when they are the ones who failed?

Growing up with no real hope of being accepted by any group taught emotional and spiritual independence. What else is there to do if I am to keep going. Being hated helped make it far easier to stick to my path. Selling out to society was not an option, since no matter what I would always be different. Being universally hated made resistance simple. What I was taught in my religion about personal worth made it easy to ignore all those trying to convince me to hate myself for being sick. What reason would I have to please such toxic people? It wouldn't get me anywhere, and would only cause me to throw away everything of value.

I am different than others, and no one will let me forget that. I have different experiences than others. I don't have the same options as others in life. Of course, I can't share the same values, interests or motivations as others, including those who claim to share my religion and were taught the same principles which they then threw away. I tend to have very little in common with others. I don't care.

One of my interests is steel. It has had a special place for me ever since I picked up a piece of metal when I was little and felt all tingly. In high school I pursued metal shop and welding. I continued studying welding in college and became a certified structural welder. For pursuing what I love I was labeled a stupid loser by my family. No interest of mine was ever acceptable, and was used against me. If I could fight to hold on to life against opposition I can hold onto interests in the face of opposition.

A long college experience was out of the question. It was hard to have much of a class load when unable to move off the floor from pain.

Welding was a physical job. Higher education was not a great option at the time I was learning to weld. A short break in the Crohn's problem came soon after I got my LA City welding license, and I was able to get a job as a welder, which brought me to San Bernardino. I loved it. My family wanted to take that away from me, and were very discouraging. They tried to convince me that I was somehow just trying to prove something by taking a physical job. They were trying to get me to doubt myself so I would give up, which they kept trying to get me to do. I was a welder because it is something I love, in a world which gives me very little to love.

Loving welding, which I did for seven years, was not enough, though. I ended up at Kaiser when the company changed insurance, and things got very difficult and out of control. Eventually I would have to stop. I had planned ahead for that eventuality. I didn't want to leave welding and steel, so I because a certified welding inspector so the physical burden would be gone but I could stay involved with what I love. I am still an inspector now. Changing jobs also got me away from Kaiser, and I was able to recover. Crohn's came close to taking away something I love.

Functioning with an active case can be challenging. It was necessary to make adjustments at times, like working on a different schedule to avoid the worst of the pain. It is necessary to have a plan in place for the problems which occur at any time.

I wasn't able to grow up with the same expectations from life as others. I had to dream within the reality of my situation. I couldn't expect life to just hand me anything I wanted. I was lucky that I started this so young, since I didn't have to have the pain of losing a life I never had, like those who develop this later in life.

I was also taught some of my most valuable lessons by lizards, of all things, when I was at a young age, probably because I grew up with an affinity to lizards since I was 3 or 4. But even Job, in all he went through, in all that was taken away, knew to ask the beasts and they will teach, if you are not so conceited in being human and supposedly a "higher" life form. One thing I was taught by lizards is that it is possible to sense when one is being focused on by someone else. Related to that was the concept of being mentally invisible to those focusing on me. It helped keep me alive. One person trying to guess my thoughts described it as like trying to read a brick wall. That was good, since he later made attempts to kill me. My mother was no better at it. Another thing lizards teach is that when other methods fail you have to be ready to drop your tail and run. Everything can be taken away, except for what I hold inside. It is best to be ready to let go, or something will be used to destroy you if you don't let go of it.

For some reason even getting a job as an inspector still made me a stupid loser and a failure. Their attempts to get me to throw away what helps me extends to everything that helps me. It is not people's intentions to have me able to function or be successful at something. That would make me independent.

I have needed consideration from employers regarding my condition. It is just a fact of living with this. Most have been at least tolerant. It also means that I have to follow every rule better than anyone else, since I am highly scrutinized and I can't give them the excuses they look for to get rid of me.

9

We have been told in my religion to stand for something. We have also been taught to do what is right regardless of any unpleasant consequences. I never had to worry about making anyone hating me, since that was independent of my actions. There has never been any opportunity to please anyone even if I had tried. I ended up with a career where I don't make friends. Perfect. This was also a career where I had to make an oath to place the public welfare above all else, with a long list of what all else means.

I don't make friends even among other inspectors, and especially not among inspectors who pretend to share my religion. I was viewed as a trouble maker. I wasn't passing bad stuff, and I wasn't letting them bully me into going along with the rampant fraud taking place among inspectors. Being half a foot shorter than I would have been (from prednisone) means that people very often think I can be intimidated. I've had to go through that since I was little and so I was well used to being treated like that, whether it was from a contractor or from other inspectors.

Retaliation was used also within a couple companies I worked for. I was ordered to lie about problems found, being told that if there is a problem I should hide it so everyone is happy. It was even more of an insult when people claiming to follow my religion jumped in and ordered me to go along with it and "accept it". That was an even worse betrayal, since I had made and know the sacred covenants and oaths they had made and thrown away, both as inspectors and a members of this religion.

On one job I had to fight them all the way to the top of the building, with management telling the contractors that everything is fine and they don't know why I am causing these problems. That building is only still standing because I stood up to them and refused to pass bad welds. There was only one inspector who didn't turn on me. He was a youth pastor for his church and they couldn't get him to violate his conscience, even at risk of losing his job. I'm a priest in my church, although I will not accept money for religious services and the rites I perform for people, so I work, but being a priest is most important. We had something in common. One thing was that there is something more important than either money or life itself. After that building I ended up working down in San Diego for a short time. I ended up working on a building just a block over from where I made my covenants, and I had that place in view as I worked. It felt good. It was also sad, because of what others had once also accepted and not went against. I continued to fight them, but the lawyers got involved and I couldn't fight them. I refused to back down, though, knowing they were getting rid of me.

This was no easy decision. I would lose some good health insurance and my treatment would be interrupted. I always have to have that on my mind, but there are more important things than life, like staying true to my path and to myself. Why would I want to be like those people? I can't share their motivations, and they will never accept mine. So what. We believe in free choice. They made theirs.

As bad as that company was, the next company I was with was even worse. They called me into a meeting one day after I had been with them for a month. It turned out that the meeting was about me and how I wasn't passing bad welds. Since I can't just fail something without giving a code section it is in violation of, they ordered me to stop caring code books with me. They ordered me to pass EVERY weld regardless of the quality. And they ended the meeting telling me that if I don't obey them they have people everywhere and they are going to "get me" no matter where I go. One person at the meeting even referenced his war record, as if that excuses deliberate fraud!. He had made the same oath I had as an inspector. Being a veteran doesn't make him any less of a traitor to the public.

Who takes an oath seriously? That is more in the realm of fiction and ideals, stories from a long time ago in a land far, far away. What about a Hippocratic Oath, or a Florence Nightingale Oath? Are people any different just because they chose a different job? The answer is no. People are just people, and no one is safe until people recognize that ranks and titles don't have anything to do with reality. Ideals are nice, but when one deceives themselves into thinking that some ideal is automatically reality, especially when discrediting any evidence otherwise, then the ideal can never be achieved since it is no longer a goal to achieve. People won't work for something they claim to already have.

10

What is help? It is easier to define what help isn't. Let's discuss that.

First of all, advice is not what people need, especially from people who haven't experienced the problem that they think they have the answer to.

Help is not help when someone is helping because they would feel bad if they didn't help. That has nothing to do with helping someone else because that means that the person is actually focused on themselves. They are doing it to make themselves feel better, not the person needing help.

Pity is not what is needed. Pity is what people offer when they don't want to do anything to change a situation. Many people in society have taken it upon themselves to be professional mourners. The rest of us have to suffer for it. Professional mourners have to have someone to mourn to keep their job…

One needs to actually listen to someone or just mind their own business if they don't want to listen. There is the story of a woman trying to work, take classes and take care of children who could have used some help. Some people decided that they would help, but wouldn't listen. The woman asked that someone help watch the children so she could do the studying she needed to do. The people who pretended to help contradicted her request, and told her that she would feel better if someone did some cleaning. In the end, it was the same as no help at all because the actual needs were not met, yet there is still the obligation of having to be grateful for nothing. They didn't go to that woman with the intention of meeting her stated needs. They went there to make themselves feel like they care, but not care enough to even listen. We don't need to be told what we need.

We are not here to make someone feel like a hero. We are not here to gratify someone's ego. We are not here to be used, which is often what is really happening when people supposedly mean well. We are not here to harm ourselves to please someone. Meaning well would mean doing something healthy and liberating, without control or coercion. Healing is related to the word "healthy", not poison. We are here to live our lives, without interference from those who don't want us to. If we are so pathetic, such inferior beings with no right to live in the world, then why do people think they need to cripple us. What are they afraid of? Themselves. The majority of supposedly spiritual people have told me that they have a problem with me not being obsessed with wealth and fame and popularity (I mean that I have literally been told that by them). Most have been greatly offended because someone tries to live with a different view of life. They haven't been able to take away the birds at midnight, or the moon setting over the ocean. I can't share with them what that means. I have no power to show them what they don't want to see. I also enjoy long walks with an IV pole around the hospital ward.

Healthy people, if they care about those who need help, need to help themselves first. They can't help if they get messed up with "caring". There is a reason for the oxygen mask instruction on a plane which say to first put your mask on before trying to help someone else get their mask on. If you pass out you aren't going to help anyone with their mask. First get yourself stable and safe. Martyrs are only good for Hollywood writers. Your "caring" doesn't save anyone if your dead. If you want to help, then don't cripple yourself, don't throw away your ability to help. You won't pull anyone up if you fall over the cliff yourself. "Caring" about others in a deeper sense means that you must care about yourself. You must love yourself (in a real sense and not just looking in a mirror and saying it) to love others in a real sense. There may be a love there for someone, but if you can't love yourself it will never come out in a meaningful way. Narcissists all hate themselves, and that is at the root of the things they do. They are very insecure, and their behaviors are overcompensation for how they see themselves but won't admit.

Maybe the most helpful thing someone can do, besides living in reality, would be to just treat people as people and stop treating people as diseases. When someone is behaving toward me differently because they find out I am sick, it is as though they are treating ME as the disease, which means I can't be included in anything. I am different, and rubbing it in my face, setting up a glass wall around me, doesn't help anything. I don't care that someone feels awkward, not knowing the "proper" protocol around a sick person. My feet are already quite numb from being stepped on, and just acting like I'm just some person won't cause me any more pain. We are more than an illness, and it would be neat for once to have that recognized, rather than being approached as an enemy to the established social order. I am not defined by an illness, but it is others who insist on defining me by it. I can't get rid of someone else's insecurities, and it is an attack when those insecurities are passed on to me as my fault for being sick. Staying out of the way can be an effective form of help.

Another side to this is the case of the other part of society which denies that someone can have a real problem if they are able to function, ignoring the extremes someone has to go to in order to function. After a lifetime of hatred, not everyone is going to show their pain on the outside. It doesn't mean it isn't there. We can be good at hiding it around predators, in order to survive. Why would we want to invite an attack? What I have is inside, and it doesn't show much on the outside, until it reaches the point that I am unable to continue. I had to grow up with good reflexes, since I would come under physical attack at any moment, being told I am just faking being sick. One thing about narcissists is that they will deny that someone else is experiencing something just because they themselves are not experiencing it. That mentality is found at all areas of society, especially including the medical professions. What pain is worse, the pain of the disease or the pain inflicted on me by others for being sick? It never matters how many surgeries I have, I'm supposedly always just faking it for attention. Lizards are very wise.

If sick people are hiding in plain sight (actually they aren't hiding they are just trying to live), why do people need to spot them? Is isolation going to help us? Do we need to be quarantined for the safety of humanity? Is it too much to ask that we be allowed to have interests that we pursue, just like other people?

There was a case a few years back regarding refugees fleeing a war. People were actually angry to see that the refugees had cell phones! Society isn't happy unless vulnerable people are completely destroyed. Can anyone see that those are people. They had their own lives like other people, and they had their world flipped over by the actions of others they had to flee. Does having a phone mean that someone can't possibly have a real problem? That is exactly what people said. Same with other homeless people who have phones. Some even have cars that they have to live in. They were once like everyone else, and something bad happened. They ended up in an unpleasant situation, but that is just a circumstance, it is not who they are. Does a society that even wants to pretend to care really seek to completely destroy those less fortunate, wanting to make sure that they are never able to rise again from the ashes of a life taken away? Victim blaming never ends and has no limit. It is those who have to endure who understand. We don't have a choice but to endure what life has handed us. But we have no obligation to accept the behavior of those who want to take away all we have if we are impudent enough to not fit whatever stereotype someone has regarding people with serious illness.

The government can offer some form of help, except that it is often a noose rather than a safety net. People are sometimes punished for even trying to overcome their disability. It isn't just the government. The government is merely an expression of the society which created it. It is not just the government. One company I worked for as an inspector had another inspector break his arm. He went on worker's comp for a time. When he was recovered enough to agree to some partial work which he could do while continuing to heal, the company decided to take the money back because they said that he could have been working in construction all along with that broken arm. Confused about why they turned on him when he was trying to do them a favor and help where he could, their response was "We have an attorney and you don't."! I got out of there, knowing that if they could do that to him they would do it to me. I had been treated nice enough for a time, but that was because I was able to do some things that the others couldn't at the time. Still, my turn was coming, and I'm glad I left when I did. Help is supposed to make things better. At least that company didn't order me to lie or make any terrorist threats against me like others.

Just because some sick person is being nice enough to let someone "help" with something, that does not entitle anyone to take over someone's life. There is a universe of difference between "back-up" and domination. One is helpful, even empowering under the right conditions, and the order is destructive and crippling. Respect for individual sovereignty and self-determination are an absolute requirement if people want to pretend to care and "help". Anything more is oppression and not healthy. The hero complex people develop is not caring, it is a psychosis. We have a principle in this religion that someone is to ask for help, and people are not to impose themselves in someone's life unless they ask for help from that person first. To do otherwise is a boundary violation and is the beginning of personal aggrandizement for the "hero".

This doesn't mean that "well" people are the only ones who do this stuff. Sick people can also be just as narcissistic and predatory when they see a chance to show their superiority over someone. Sometimes, those people can be even worse, looking even harder for someone to bash down and scapegoat for all their frustrations in life, since they didn't get the opportunity to show their superiority to the general population. Some sick people can be very inconsiderate of other people's problems, even though you would think that going through what they went through might have taught them some empathy. Some of those I have known have spoken against the genocide of their particular pet group they favor, yet have no problem with genocide when it is against another group. Experience is not an indication of learning, and age is not an indication of perception. Age makes people old. Learning makes people wise. There is no direct relation between the two.

There have been MANY narcissists I have met with problems, who have used those problems for entitlement, which becomes license to treat other people any way they want. Abuse and victimizing and committing crimes against people is not necessarily unusual for this particular group, and they have given their problems as the excuse why they are entitled to do such things to anyone they want. They also attack anyone with a worse problem, usually with the claim that the person must be faking it for attention, since they see someone with an actual disability as competition for attention, which narcissists claim an exclusive right to. They engage in victim blaming just like the rest of society, except that they don't apply it to themselves for some reason. There are many out there who do a real good job of trying to prove that having a problem does not automatically make someone an *innocent* victim of circumstance. Fortunately, narcissists only make up somewhere around 5% of the population, depending on which study you look at.

I have known a small number, especially ones in my church more so than out in general society, who have gone pretty far to prove certain political parties right about disabled people and milking the system. It is unfortunate that those people do actually exist, although they are the exception rather than the rule. They are helping to give a bad name to people who do have a problem, and are encouraging the attitudes toward such people with problems. I have known people who have refused to do anything to help their problems, and even do things to prevent the problem from being helped. There are numerous narcissistic people I have known who had been prescribed medications for their problem yet refuse to take it, and will continued to whine to people about their problem that they refused to do anything about even though they were given help. They even lie and say they can't get the medication they already have but refuse to take. Some even cry about how they are trying to get that same medication they already have in their house but it is being refused, and so on. I have known people who only got on assistance so they can do drugs all the time without having to worry about losing a job. I have seen many other things as well, and there are resources being withheld from people struggling with illness. Narcissists will whine and cry about how no one will help them, yet refuse the help they were pretending to beg for, and still go on crying about how no one will help them, with all the ridiculous over-acting and facial contortions they practice in a mirror.

We have all run into those people at gas stations who ask for money for gas for their car, yet refuse when one offers to give them gas, with them insisting that they be given the money instead of the gas they said they needed. It is no different.

There are also many hypochondriacs out there, besides the people who are legitimately sick. There are people who fake it for attention, quite often narcissists. There are also the narcissists who engage in the Munchausen by proxy stuff and both make and keep people sick when they would not have been otherwise. There are people who get pain killers when they are not in pain (I've known some who claim pain but use those drugs recreationally when they are not in pain.) There are doctors OK with fraud who keep those people supplied, and the selfishness of those people abusing such things makes it so that people who are in intense pain can't get help since everyone who claims to be in serious pain is looked at like a drug addict who needs help withheld (for our own good supposedly). The honest are not able to get a break from the pain, which can reach dangerous, indeed deadly, intensity. Sick people are the ones who have to pay for the sins of the others.

I am sure we all know those people who are not disabled who like to park in handicapped parking spots, taking those spots away from those who need them. Inconveniencing disabled people doesn't seem to matter to those people who only want to save a matter of seconds of walking. I have also known those who will misuse their spouse's handicapped tag so they can get away with it, and who didn't even care at all when the spouse warned them that the tag would be revoked if they got caught and then the disabled spouse would no longer be able to use the handicapped parking spaces. Those non-disabled people don't care what the effects are on the others they are stealing from.

There are also those sick people who have the same heart and mind of the ruling cliques, and are just like them, discriminating against anyone perceived to be weak, and they see no hypocrisy in discriminating against people with a problem. Experience does not teach empathy, since that would have to be a choice, and it requires setting aside all the hubris and conceit in order to place people on an equal level. There are sick narcissists also, who deny that anyone else has a problem since that would be competition for "sympathy". They complain about the ruling cliques only when they are not the ruler of the clique. They use sickness as a tool to get what they want, and it becomes a weapon, just as those not sick can use health as a weapon.

We have a society that creates both predator and prey. Both are necessary for the other to exist. What if there is another way? What if people just stop playing that society game? It exists as an artificial construct entirely in the minds of those who agree it exists – what they call an objectified reality. What if people quit listening to the piper? Why did they even ever listen at all? Are they just drones? Those are the real sick people, they just don't know it yet since they haven't been scapegoated by the society they sold out to.

11

Abuse of any sort can't exist without a whole army of people in society ready to enforce it and protect it at every turn without question. This even includes the medical professions, besides all elements of society. There is no group that the problem doesn't exist in. Eradicating it would require a new society, or no society at all (not necessarily a bad thing, not through violence, of course, but through changing people's hearts, which is the only way to have real change). To have either means the current society would have to die if it is to be reborn. It is not limited to religious groups. It wasn't created by religious groups. It exists in all areas of society, commercial, civil, government, and anywhere where there are people, because the problem is created by people and exists within the people. When incidents make national news, it is only an expression of the American society that allows and upholds such things, and therefore also a collective expression of the individuals who make up that society. The United States is run by a grope-ocracy at state and federal levels where there is no accountability, and the people who do such things are even praised, with sexual assaulting someone almost seeming to be a requirement to be elected. Laws are being enforced by people with no accountability, answering to no one but the KKK they serve, and protected from prosecution for their crimes by the Wall of Silence and by powerful unions who can suppress any complaints. Power has been given to the wrong people, yet they are merely an expression of the society who elected them. It is not limited to one political party no matter what news network you want to listen to exclusively in rejection of all others. Tuning out the other voice only makes someone part of the problem, no matter which side one happens to be on, since sides are part of the problem, making everything in society a team sport with no more to do with making a better world than a game of ping-pong. One should look at the #METOO movement to see how it pervades every part of society as a whole without exception. It is not an exclusive problem of one business or profession. I only mentioned my profession in this because this book is sharing my personal experience, but I have seen it everywhere, and so has everyone else. It is not a problem of one gender, sexual orientation, or a problem of any other segment of society people want to separate, isolate and destroy. One group can't be scapegoated for what they all do regardless of the "noble" pretensions of such groups doing the blaming, which most often is simply hypocrisy. Choosing a scapegoat is part of the problem, since it allows people to focus on one group only and ignore the bigger picture. It is a distraction from the problem, a mere decoy, allowing the general population to pretend that the problem doesn't exist within them. Therefore, people are able to get away with such crimes, since to blame one only is to approve of what the others are doing. Double standards. The problem is among all the people who try to enforce the "Everything is just fine, nothing to see here, so shut up about what we are doing to you" attitude. One day I might not be standing alone, but that is only dreaming.

I have worked with convicted killers during my occupation, where I have worked in various prisons. I have felt safer there than in a church building. I mean it literally. Convicted killers are far more respectful, too. Even gangsters have a form of honor, and I have seen entire church congregations without any.

There were two of the leaders who were willing to protect us, and refused to force us to give up our son. The spy network in that church would give word any time there was a change in leaders. We had to stay on top of it and warn the new leaders, since they would be contacted about forcing us to give up our son within days. The women leaders went along with the campaign of terror and supported all attempts to destroy us. So, the women especially, although not exclusively, spread every lie they could about us to get people to hate us for not giving up our son. Most of the women I met in leadership positions throughout my whole life were and are narcissists, and people mistake shameless self-promotion and jockeying as piety and devotion, with the rest of the women happy to just sit there passively and stare at a wall rather than stand against the things going on (most especially the ones who were converts who had come from certain other religious groups, which is a huge percentage of them). So, I had to face the constant lies about having affairs (actually the people accusing me of that including my mother and Amy's mother were the ones having affairs as well as a number of the people on their side), and there was the constant accusation that our son is not ours but we "stole" him. Much of the abuse was directed at Amy since she had less ability to resist them. This stuff went against everything that those people claimed to believe is right, the bogus pretended principles that they are willing to speak one day a week but go against the other six days. They tried to use intimidation at me at church, but whispering to me every week "I've been talking to your mother" has less impact when you have received direct death threats at church. (The sentence of death has never been revoked either.) I don't go to church for those people, I go there in spite of them. I have to hear how "righteous" certain people are, and of course how ungrateful and evil I am for not giving in to something unconscionable. It is strange that no matter what principles people profess, people won't stand up for what is right, yet will always stand up for what is wrong. They can't claim ignorance of the beliefs they profess. They know the truth of the matter, and have had all facts before them. They did not choose their sides in ignorance. According to their own stated beliefs their treason against what is right places them outside of forgiveness, just like they placed me, not that I need their forgiveness for standing up for what is right. They declared, as is stated, that the sun is not shining at noon day. There is nothing that can be done to help people who know the truth and have chosen such evil with their eyes open to it. There is no fact that they can be given which they don't already have, and have even admitted to be true. None of it was a misunderstanding. It is blasphemy for them to claim to have the Spirit of Truth and to fight what they know to be true, but they know that.

I know of no other case like mine where someone has gone through these things without leaving the religion. I don't judge a religion by those who don't follow it. I got it for myself and they can't take it away from me. It doesn't help the feeling of betrayal that all the people who have gone through this stuff feel when sometimes in the world wide conferences of the church some leaders will comment that people are leaving over "petty" little nonsense things, or meaningless little grudges they just need to get over. Murder is not petty, especially when people don't stop wanting someone dead. Child molestation is not petty. The abuse people go through, often fully sanctioned by the people of the church, is not petty. The betrayal people face when they try to get help to save their lives is not petty. When the people committing these crimes are protected from consequences, that is betrayal and indicates a serious cancer within which will destroy the whole body.

I am not the one cursing them, or cursing my family. They cursed themselves through their own free will choices and the only way to bring honor is to stand against their evil. This isn't about seeking to harm or get back at them. This is about speaking up to try to save some innocent victims, and to try to prevent innocent people from being harmed by predators. It is not about the past, because these things never stopped. This is not about revenge. This is about keeping blood off of my hands. This isn't about me not "letting go". I have been trying to go and they are the ones won't let me go. It isn't wrong to do what is right. Is it right to save, or to destroy? You get one choice.

It is not those who speak up who are making the church look bad. It is the people who commit such crimes against the people who make it look bad. The only way to redemption is to take a stand and call things what they are. People get away with it by using such bogus pseudo-religious sounding ideas as loving the sinner, which means hating the victims of their action. One can't look the other way without being guilty. What about loving the victims? Does anyone care enough to defend the victims from the abuse? When will the victims receive love? Are the victims not worthy of love? Obviously not to them. If you don't stand and say "This is wrong" then you are saying that it is right and approve of it, even in silence. I have a sticker on the computer I am using to type this, related to my work as an inspector, which says "Silence is the voice of complicity". To defend evil is to purposely allow it to continue. No one is ever being a "peacemaker" by demanding that the innocent march themselves off to the gas chamber. Destroying lives is never peace. Why is peace denied to the victims? This kind of attitude exists everywhere in society, not just this church or other churches. To change this takes people not being such cowards. It is said that evil wins when good people do nothing, so the victory of evil is nearly 100%. It will take people who will not bow down to intimidation, no matter how much people say that we "have the greater sin" for holding people accountable. We already have had it explained to us constantly that we are so evil that God is punishing us, and being born with a major illness proves it to the world. We have heard all our lives how we deserve everything done to us, including murder. The sentence of death was not just pronounced against me, it was also explained to me by others that death is what I deserve. People still don't think I got the message clearly enough. We all know we are "not perfect either". We have been reminded of how evil we supposedly have always been since we were born. We need people with a conscience, and willing to follow it. So what if they condemn me to hell for speaking the truth that they all know to be true. A hell of human beings is better than a heaven of devils. They already have tried to bring down hell on every aspect of my life, simply because a narcissist ordered them to do such things to me and to countless others who have had to flee for their lives.

What they were doing and the effects from it was great testimony to the benefit of the principles claimed but rejected. Just look at what happens when people don't follow those principles. But I alone can't bring any credit to the church when the people of the church are bringing such dishonor to it.

Trying to save people from predators is not being hateful. It is about loving the innocent who are being destroyed. Holding people accountable is not being unforgiving or unmerciful. It is about choosing what is right over what is wrong. It is having mercy on the people who are being hurt. I have had a number of surgeries where parts of my intestines were cut out. Does that mean that I hate my intestines so much? It was to save the rest of my intestines and save my life that the sections killing me (they brought me to the brink of death) had to be removed. It is about saving, not about having any intention to destroy.

Anyway, I was given a position of giving some lessons to a group of other priests. I reluctantly agreed, knowing that there is a serious danger in a spotlight with these people. Then, an even more serious mistake was made. I asked someone for help, due to a worsening flare-up.

Once again, there was a disease surrounding me which is worse than the one inside me.

12

In 2019, symptoms started getting worse at the end. There was a noticeable difference in the foods I could tolerate. Early 2020 it was getting bad, and eventually I had to go back to my old stand-by milk diet, which was working. I had ended back at Kaiser. Things always get out of control when I'm at Kaiser, and this time was no different.

In the Spring of 2020, I contacted my gastroenterologist about the worsening flare-up. This was when his narcissistic behaviors began to be manifest. I showed a weakness. That was his cue to harm me. He started by virtually ignoring me. I was on Stelara and Thalidomide, but only minimal doses of those. Stelara was every two months, but it only had an effect for one month. So I would be symptom free for one month, and then the symptoms would intensify over the next month, often with vomiting toward the end of the bad month. What made things worse was that this doctor used the Stelara as a weapon, and there would be a long delay before I could get it. I would spend weeks trying to get it. The pharmacy would send refill requests which would not be filled, since the doctor would tell me that there are already refills available. The reality was that he wasn't placing refills on the prescriptions, and so the pharmacy couldn't refill it. He would ignore the pharmacy requests and it could take weeks of asking before I could get it again. That extra delay made my symptoms even more severe than they had to be. Then the good month was only partially symptom free.

During the summer of 2020, my condition was getting quite bad. The vomiting had set in now. I asked for help since I wasn't being helped by the doctor who seemed intent on letting me die.

There had been a shuffle of leaders in the church early in that year. Unfortunately, these leaders were the opposite of the two who had chosen to help protect us. A new batch of Sneetches got stars on their bellies.

I asked for and was blessed by a couple people from the church in the summer. One of them was one of the new leaders. I don't remember the words of the blessing. I do remember what happened a couple hours after.

I had made a mistake and showed a weakness to predators. That was their cue to strike.

I received a call from that leader. He launched into an attack. He told me that I was teaching false doctrine and going against what the church says. The irony was that I hadn't chosen any of the lessons, he did. It wasn't my doctrine. Everything I quoted came from the leaders of the church and were found in lesson manuals. What he was most angry about was some unpleasant historical facts mentioned in the history of the church. The church doesn't deny any of it, and it is even taught in lesson manuals published by the church education department and is common knowledge. This leader ordered me to lie about it since it isn't nice. Unfortunately, that stuff actually happened and it has to be acknowledged, as bad as it was. I refused to lie. I'm obviously the only person who takes things seriously enough to look. But the historical incident involved was because of a very destructive narcissist early in the history of this church who did much damage, especially to her own children as well as damage to the church. It is a fact about narcissists that they back up other narcissists, especially against the victims. The narcissist leader who was now trying to cause me harm was backing up the historical narcissist and approved of what that narcissist did to destroy her own family as well as harm as many people in the church as she could. Of course a narcissist sees nothing wrong with destroying people.

I won't go into great detail about the doctrinal matters involved in this church as that is outside the scope of this book, and would more properly be the subject of another book. I will keep it relevant to the subject of this book.

In August of 2020, I was working in 120 degree heat near Blythe, CA. I was late getting medication as usual, so this particular week was extra bad and the vomiting worse, which resulted in extreme dehydration. I had to go to the emergency room. By the time I made it there I was in a full body cramp unable to move. I was admitted.

A scan showed an ileus, of course, which I already knew. I was given fluid and steroids, which brought things under control. I was then symptom free again. I was released, and spent a week recovering. It was a good week without problems. I even got the Stelara. But there was another problem which wasn't addressed or even mentioned at the time, which had also shown up in the scan.

A week after I had been released, my colon perforated. The dehydration had impacted my colon. It had shown up in the scan, but no one said or did anything about that, and it could have been treated then before the intestine died. But nothing was said or done while there was still a chance. If I had been told I could have done something even if they wouldn't.

I went back into the emergency room, where my pain was mocked. My intestines had ruptured, but for some reason that just made me a crybaby faking it for attention. A scan showed the rupture, and then surgery was performed. I was in a medically induced coma for a couple days. I woke up with a colostomy bag.

That added a new dimension to my problems. Losing almost all but maybe four or five inches of colon then produced difficulty absorbing water. My weight dropped from 165 to 116 quickly. My gastroenterologist continued to ignore me.

Previously in the year, that friend from long ago had turned on us, and was trying to break us up, and the lying crossed some serious red lines that can't just be re-crossed. I wouldn't take it. So I prayed about it and the answer was to leave that toxic person. I didn't tell Amy about it or about the gaslighting that person was engaging in to try to get me to leave Amy. I wasn't going to take the lying anymore. But, I wasn't going to say anything to Amy until after Amy saw it from herself and came to the same conclusion on her own without any influence from me.

It was a great relief not to be getting constant lies and flipped stories from that person any more. I only put up with it as long as I had to. I was pretty sick of hearing genocide being justified. That person had been a traitor before with a rather murderous disposition, and that person proved that they hadn't changed. That person threw away every chance they were given until there were no more chances to give. I was pretty sick of being treated as just a piece of their personal property, which is the only way that narcissists like them treat people. And like all other narcissists, this one followed the principle of trying to destroy anything or anyone they can't own.

That person found out about my surgery, and being a predator decided to strike while I was having a moment of weakness. That person went after Amy and used the same gaslighting on her, as well as other tactics. One of the tactics that person used was to give a message to me that the person was in contact with people who had promised to come back some day to kill me, including the one who said he would kill me with Crohn's disease. That person also said they were going to tell my mother about my condition, knowing that my mother wants me dead. Amy's family also found out, and so they also decided that this was the time to strike.

Amy prayed about that person also, and did come to the same conclusion that it was not possible to continue a friendship with someone out to destroy us. Only after Amy told me did I share what that person was telling me about Amy to try to get me to hate Amy.

The first few weeks after the surgery were very hard. I went off of Stelara at the request of the surgeon, so that it wouldn't interfere with healing. I stayed on Thalidomide, which was the more important one.

Even though I had lost much weight, with much of that weight being from dehydration, in a short time I was able to gain back 20 pounds. I have been loaded up on enough steroids that I had no dietary restrictions. I could at least swallow anything, even though I wouldn't be able to absorb plant material. I had a diet with 60 grams of fiber a day, which I considered to be a normal diet. Most of that was waste, but fiber doesn't have to be absorbed to do its job. I was recovering slowly and adjusting to the new difficulties.

A serious difficulty was the frequency of having to empty my bag. At times it could be every 10 minutes. This would happen at any time day or night, which restricted both activity and sleep. When my bag would fill up I might have a minute or less to empty it. I had to be hyper-vigilant when trying to sleep or my bag would blow. That meant that I had very little sleep, even when the output was low, since I would never know. There would be no warning when things would go from quiet to blasting out a gallon in an hour.

<h1 style="text-align:center">13</h1>

At one point a home health nurse thought that the surgical wound could possibly be infected. The brand of bags I was being provided by the insurance were really bad for my particular case. Other people have great luck with them, but I had complications. They were a very expensive and well promoted brand, but they wouldn't bond to my skin or seal. The hydrocolloid wax base would stay stiff and would not follow the contour of my abdomen around the surgical wound and the scar crease from a previous bowel resection. It would pull away from my skin. When I went back to working I found the plastic the bags were made of would spontaneously develop holes. The bags would just fall off onto the floor, making exercising tricky and I had to modify exercises to keep from breaking the bag. Other people have a great time with those bags and no problem, but it didn't work out for me. The seal would break up to 5 times a day, and the insurance was only allowing me to have 20 per month. The bag was very close to the surgical wound, which had openings left for drainage due to the contamination of the abdominal cavity from the perforation. So, stool from my bag would leak into those openings multiple times a day and it was difficult to clean those holes. I went to the emergency room as advised by the nurse to get it checked out for infection.

At the emergency room, a surgeon checked the wound. There was no infection found. Unfortunately, in order to check for infection and clean everything out properly, I had to be re-opened. The wound had been scarring over nicely and on schedule, beginning from the lower part of the wound. That part that was completely scarred was left as is, and gave proof that it was healing. Now my wound was opened to about an inch wide for the remainder of the wound. It was not a pleasant sight. When the surgeon looked at it and told them to give me a pain killer, I knew it was not going to be fun. He ripped me open. He, as a surgeon, was probably used to looking at stuff like that, but I definitely did not need to see what I looked like on the inside. The inside of a person is quite ugly compared to the outside and I'm glad that stuff is normally covered up with skin. I've always been unconscious when open.

Now I had an inch wide wound with only several deep sutures to keep my abdominal cavity from opening completely. There was nothing now to hold my abdominal muscles in place, and I was told that it was pretty much guaranteed that I would have a hernia soon.

It was decided by this surgeon to try a wound vacuum. An air-tight dressing was put on, and the vacuum set up, which would such away any fluid leaking from the wound. It is something which has good success in some cases for speeding healing. There was a problem with my case, though.

Great idea, except that the dressing for the wound vacuum overlapped the bag. Now, instead of stool leaking a little into the wound, the problem was now vacuum powered, sucking stool into the wound. Nothing like mechanizing a problem to take it to a new level. We didn't have enough supplies to change the vacuum dressing and lines. It would only be useable for one day at the best, usually only a few hours, and then it couldn't be used. So it did nothing to help me.

I had a post-surgical follow up appointment with the surgeon who removed my colon. It had been a few weeks since the surgery. He looked at the wound and commented that I was healing well, as demonstrated by the section that had scarred over already. He agreed that the wound vacuum was not working out, especially with the lack of supplies to keep it running. I was also very dehydrated due to only absorbing maybe 20% of the fluid I drink, often less. The rest was coming out in my bag. The surgeon ordered me to be admitted to the hospital so they could come up with a solution to the high ostomy output. Also during this visit the surgeon commented about the impacted colon and discussed the scan with me. It was dehydration that caused me to lose my colon. I don't have proof that he didn't inform my gastroenterologist, but it is known that the gastroenterologist had been consulted about my condition at the time but was ignoring me.

One thing about that gastroenterologist is that every doctor who saw his name in my file warned me about how he treats people. It wasn't just patients he treated so awful, but he treated other doctors the same way. Doctors don't normally say things like that about another doctor. It was every doctor who got involved in my case who warned me about him.

Back in the hospital. The nurses were almost all pathological liars. That made things very difficult. They were making stuff up like I don't know anything. They would rather make up nonsense than look something up. One of the incidents involved food. I had been put on a regular diet and had a meal after I was admitted. The next day, my meal was delivered to the unit, but numerous hours went by. I asked about it, and the nurses (more than one) told me that I had been ordered NPO and that must be the reason I didn't get the food, with them claiming that the food service never sent anything because I was NPO. I talked to the food service and they looked in the record and I was still ordered on a regular diet, which they had sent. The nurses flat out refused to check the order. When I brought up that I had been given a meal already when I was admitted, a nurse said something very shockingly stupid, shocking even to someone who hears nothing but made up stupidity. The nurse told me that sometimes they give someone a regular meal right before they go NPO! They insisted that no meal had been sent for me. If it is not safe for someone to eat they don't give them food. Since the nurses were flat out directly refusing to check the diet order from the doctor, Amy called the doctor and the doctor had to order them to hand me my food! Guess what? Had the food really not been sent? They were lying about that too. When they were ordered to give it to me, it was the tray with my name on it which was sitting right at the door to my room, which I had been staring at the whole time. They knew it was for me the whole time, since it had my name on it, so the just grabbed it and gave it to me! That was only one of the incidents, and EVERY TIME there was any question of any nature about anything they would make up ridiculous lies. That was on top of the contempt they had for what I was going through, and supposedly I am just a retard who knows nothing about Crohn's disease and I just need to shut up and accept it!. There is no surprise that there are so many serial killers who are nurses. A large proportion of these nurses are narcissists, including Amy's family. They seem to enjoy watching people suffer. It was most extreme at Kaiser than other places, although the contempt for people was also quite noticeable at Loma Linda. It was different at Cedars-Sinai.

It was the same at the time of the surgery. Nurses also seemed to have contempt for my bag, and would deliberately jerk on the bag, which would break the seal and spill stool, every time I let a nurse touch it. I would say it is leaking, and they would deny it, and while denying the stool leaking all over, wouldn't even look at it to see if I was right. They would just deny that it was leaking stool all over and tell me I'm wrong, telling me that it is fluid leaking from my JP line, without even turning their heads to see. I would have to insist over and over again that it is stood before they would eventually turn their heads and see. They had been refusing to even look, keeping their heads turned as they ripped my bags off as if that would allow them to claim they didn't know it was happening. And, it was every time! I had to stop allowing nurses to touch my bag. They seemed completely incapable of learning anything, but then again, that would require caring. It was all the nurses. It was every subject, anytime.

While in the hospital, nothing was done to figure out why I was having so much trouble absorbing fluids. After so many days went by being on intravenous fluids, which helped the dehydration, they declared me better and sent me home. When I asked what to do about the high output they just said to take some Imodium! Did they really think that after about 40 years of having Crohn's Disease I would never have heard of Imodium? According to the nurses, that is exactly what they think. They gave me some liquid Imodium in the hospital, which was so awful I had to ask for a pill instead. They were only giving me the standard 2 mg dose, but the liquid was becoming unbearable and nauseating. The nurse I talked to then decided to make up another lie. She told me that the pharmacy doesn't carry pills. Yes they do. Then she told me that, well, the 2 mg dose only exists in liquid form and that is why they can't give me the pill instead. I couldn't believe she thought I would be that stupid that after spending my life on Imodium I wouldn't know that the pills are the same 2 mg dose and there is no other dose. They give me more than one liquid thing, they could give me more than one pill also, just like when they combine any other pills to get to the right dose. (I later discovered that being unable to do first grade math is a problem at Kaiser, and not just with nurses). She refused to look it up or talk to the doctor, as always. I'm glad that these nurses didn't decide to become doctors or there would be no chance of survival for anyone. They do so much damage within their scope of work, they are definitely not people who should be making important decisions, since they are incapable of just looking at a computer screen and refuse to verify information. There are already so many doctors like that.

I went home as ordered. I was no longer having the benefit of the steroids, and they had sent me home actively vomiting. It was not just the Crohn's problem, but it takes time for the body to adjust to such drastic changes in function. That doesn't help dehydration. The vomiting was getting better, though. I was on my own to try to figure out how to survive.

The wound, which was not being held together, kept ripping further open, eventually reaching several inches wide, with the muscles moving to my sides, with a big knot of muscles settling directly under my stoma and bag. Even the deep sutures ripped.

14

The narcissists used this opportunity to strike again. While in the hospital, I was sent a card by Amy's family. It was rather insulting that they thought they could buy my favor with that tactic after all they did and after them wanting me dead for so long. They said that they just love me so much and want me better! That's how stupid they think I am that I would forget who they are and what they want to do to me and Amy and our son. They were some of the people literally cheering for my death, and now they just love me so much?

The way that tactic works is that it was timed to try to make it appear that what they decided to do would look like they were just doing it because of how much they care about me. So what did they do? They called Adult Protective Services. The accusations they made included that I was losing weight and was starving to death, not because I had just had a major surgery on my digestive tract but because Amy refused to cook for me! This was just a continuation of when Amy's family had been doing all her life, with the whole bad daughter, bad sister, bad wife thing. I'm independent. I was able to move around freely without help, and I was not bedbound and unable to just get up and eat like that social worker had been told. I don't even need anyone to cook for me and I prefer to do that myself. I had refused to punish Amy long ago when they commanded me to for a very closely similar accusation, so they were sending in the mercenaries. The other accusation was that I was soaked in urine. The investigator found the accusations to be bogus, of course. This wasn't about loving or caring about me, it was simply to cause us as much harm as they could, just like when her family made accusations repeatedly to CPS. The card was just a set up to make them look innocent, when it was actually sent at the time they made the call to APS. The card was an attack.

They weren't the only narcissists to strike at a moment of weakness. That gastroenterologist also struck.

Prior to this moment, the gastroenterologist had told me that he was ordering a colonoscopy and endoscopy, after I had been continuing to try to get help for the flare-up which was still not being addressed. Things weren't being done about the Crohn's flare-up that he had been denying I had, even though it had shown up in the scan before the surgery. He ordered the prep, which we got from the pharmacy. Some time went by, and I wasn't seeing the colonoscopy on scheduled. I was barely able to whisper at the time due to damage from the breathing tube at the time of the surgery. It took a month and a half to get my voice back. So, Amy called the Gastroenterology department to find out when the procedure was scheduled. The gastroenterology department told her that the doctor had canceled it "because the surgery fixed the problem." That gastroenterologist had been fixated on Colitis. Every time I would talk to him he would talk about Colitis, which I didn't have. I have a long medical record and none of it says that I have Colitis. He knew that my problem is Crohn's Disease in the small intestine, but that is the way narcissists operate. They simply make stuff up to contradict people, because they have this need to show that they are the only ones who can ever be right about something. It is an instinct of theirs to contradict anyone and contradict the known facts. It is purely toddlerish oppositional behavior. He clearly had no intention of treating me. Amy was upset by what he was doing to me, so she filed a complaint, very rightfully, since the doctor was purposely keeping me sick.

I got a phone call from that doctor. He began yelling at me about the complaint. He was using this opportunity while I was almost completely unable to communicate. He ended it with declaring that I wasn't healing, and it had to be the Thalidomide preventing healing. He didn't even see me in person or look at anything, he just declared that I wasn't healing. He ignored also the fact that I had gained back 20 pounds an several weeks after bottoming out after the surgery. This stuff he was claiming was also in contradiction to what the surgeon who actually met with me and looked at the wound said. He declared that he was taking me off of Thalidomide. He was willing to put me back on Stelara, but Thalidomide was the one that was doing the most for me and so that is the one he targeted.

It didn't take long before there were problems. The Stelara would only have an effect for about three days without the Thalidomide. I stopped gaining weight right away. Within a month, other symptoms began showing, such as food not breaking down in my intestines at all. That meant that I had to restrict my diet again. Whatever is going through whole obviously is a danger. It started with only certain plant based foods, but in time eventually included all plants. Even juice wouldn't break down, and it would still be juice when it reached my bag. Animal products like milk and meat still broke down as fine as always. At this point my intestines hadn't narrowed down to the level of obstruction as before I had the steroids around the time of the surgery. Things were still passing through, even if there was zero digestion of the plant based stuff. When I would see something come through whole I would eliminate it from my diet. I was still trying to maintain a certain fiber intake, but that eventually got tricky. At this time, and for a long time after, I would still be able to eat some wheat, when I was able to eat solid food. Wheat is always the last plant I have problems with.

Thalidomide did more for me than just treat the Crohn's problem. It also kept my heart from being tachycardic. Along came that problem, with my heart feeling like it was trying to bash itself apart. That had to be addressed. Thalidomide was originally developed as a sedative, and works great for that. I need that for the severe insomnia, and going off of it meant I was back to getting 2 hours of sleep or less. That made functioning in any capacity more difficult.

Thalidomide also had been keeping the ostomy output lower than it was after. Even though I was only absorbing a small amount of fluid, that got noticeably worse after I was taken off of Thalidomide. The Stelara would only work for a few days. I would get much higher absorption during those few days, up to maybe half of what I drink, but then the absorption would drop to a very low level. Stelara was worthless without the Thalidomide, and the output got worse from the lower absorption. That was all fine with the gastroenterologist, who continued not only to deny that I have a problem, but also began even denying that I even had a problem before now. He kept up the Colitis crap. He kept telling me there was no evidence of a flare-up, in contradiction to actual test results (i.e. calprotectin levels around 650 combined with a high C-reactive protein level and high sedimentation rate). He denied the scan that showed the inflammation before the surgery.

Without the Thalidomide, the consistency of the stood went toward just pure liquid. It got to the point that so much of it was unabsorbed water that it would actually flush the bag clean. This point was reached several months after stopping the Thalidomide.

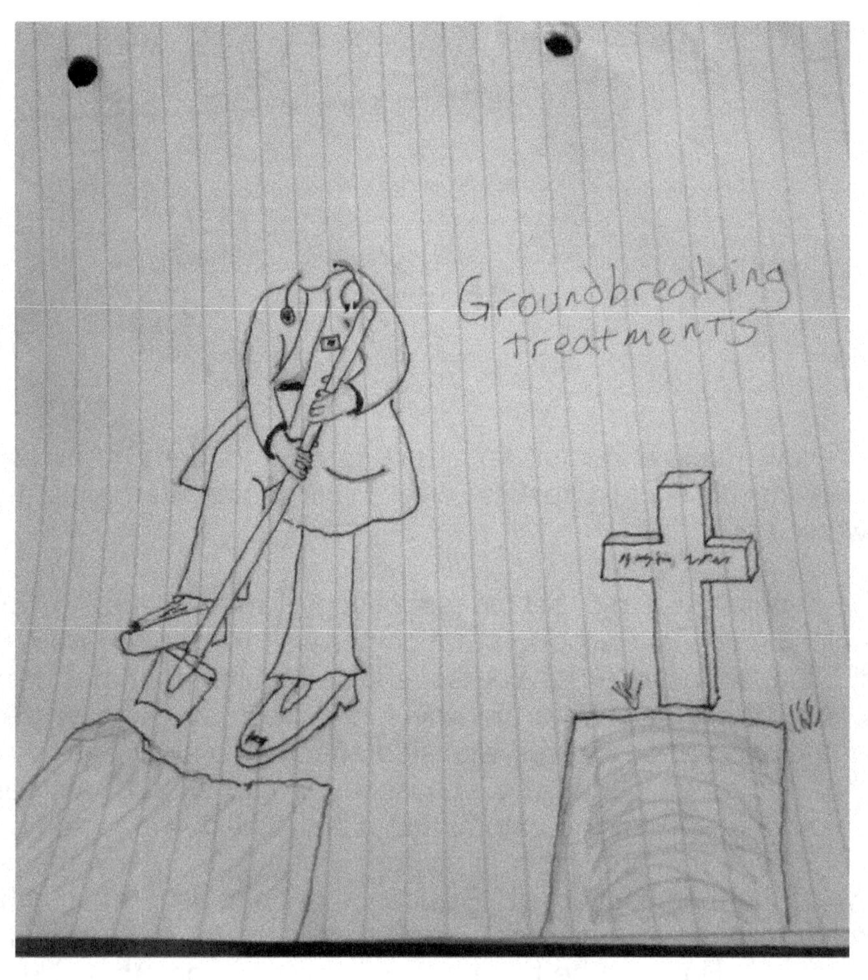

Groundbreaking
treatments

15

How does a doctor fake test results to deny a problem that is showing up on test results? Well, this gastroenterologist had that all worked out.

Eventually, I did get an endoscopy, and still had to argue for a colonoscopy, even though that doctor was refusing to treat me without it. The endoscopy, of course showed nothing. It has been only a couple times in my life that there has been anything in my stomach, and those sores resolved with little attention in short time. An odd thing that happened during the endoscopy was that the gastroenterologist said he looked for the ostomy but didn't find it! The location on the left portion of my abdomen is stated repeatedly in my medical record which he had looked at. Besides that, people I meet who are not medical professionals see the bag through my clothes and recognize what it is. How can he have honestly missed something like that which can't be hidden?

It took close to 5 months to get him to let me have the colonoscopy that he said was necessary if I wanted to be treated. He was still yelling at me about the complaint 5 months later, but in person this time, and he warned me that I "better not complain." Of course, the colonoscopy did not show anything in the several inches of colon I have left. Colonoscopies don't show anything, since the damaged small intestine is too far up from the colon. But that was known, since the scan before the surgery had shown the location clearly. The location has been known since 1997 and hasn't moved. He knew that. He was specifically looking where he knew there was no disease, and of course, repeated the lie that nothing is wrong because I don't have any sign of <u>Colitis</u>. The surgeon had noted during the surgery that there was no sign of Colitis in my colon, and that had not been the problem. But the surgeon was also not denying that I have Crohn's disease.

I knew that the endoscopy and colonoscopy were not being done to find anything, since that would not be possible through such methods. I agreed to do it because the gastroenterologist was refusing my treatment and insisted that I had to do it to get treated. I was just jumping through the hoops he set up since I didn't have a choice.

He also had some radiography done. The first incident in early 2021 involved what he had told me would be a full GI series. I had insisted on it being a full GI series, since the known bad area of active disease was so far down from my stomach. When I went in for the test, they had me drink the barium as usual, and had me roll around for a few minutes to coat my stomach. They took the picture of my stomach, with only a little barium reaching the beginning of my intestines since it had only been a matter of minutes. They told me the test was done. I asked them to check the order again, which they did. The gastroenterologist had ordered them to check my stomach only.

The gastroenterologist called me after the test and told me that there is nothing wrong with my intestines, no sign of disease, because there was nothing in my *stomach*. I confronted him about ordering them to look at my stomach only when it was supposed to be a full GI series. He played dumb and denied it. He insisted that he had ordered a full GI series, which was a lie since I had them re-check the order. He couldn't fight the fact, so he agreed to order a full GI series.

That went very similarly, but with a new twist. When I went in for that test, they confirmed that the order was for a full GI series, and they would keep taking pictures until the barium reached my bag. That sounded correct. A very short time into the test, reaching only the beginning of my small intestines in the area covered by the endoscopy and known to be clear of disease, the technician then mentioned a note in the order that they were supposed to contact the doctor when they reached that point. They called the doctor and he ordered them to *stop the testing* right then. Once again, he had prevented the bad area from being seen. He called me after that and told me again that there was no disease found and so I don't have a problem! I confronted him again about what he did to sabotage the test. He was refusing to look at the area known to have active disease. The lengths he went to so as to avoid the known disease area is an admission that he knew it was there. He was using a basic narcissist tactic that they use to try to play dumb about what they know to be true. He was as bad as the nurses, but he had more power to destroy and let people die.

From then on, in every conversation, he would repeat over and over again in the same conversation "I don't know why you don't feel well." That same line over and over again, interspersed with statements that there is no evidence I have Crohn's disease, and repeating stuff about Colitis, of which there was no sign of. Blood test results and stool calprotectin results were also denied.

Here, for contrast, I will mention what happens when someone who is not a narcissist makes a small mistake, and then fixes it. I asked a doctor for a B12 injection prescription, since I have zero absorption of it and have had to give myself injections for many years. The doctor gave me an injection right then, and it was double the usual dose. Then the doctor had me go immediately to the lab to have the levels checked. That was done in reverse order. When I got the call that the levels weren't bad, I mentioned that I had a very large dose of it right before the test. So, instead of denying what happened, instead of launching into some ridiculous medical word salad to make me think I'm too stupid to know my case and contradict a doctor-god, that doctor actually ordered a new test. This test was not immediately when the levels were still higher, but in a month when my levels would drop to an accurate baseline. I got the test at that time, and rather than the doctor denying the test result and insisting that I'm still wrong, the doctor gave me the prescription for the B12 injection! It was shocking that this was a Kaiser doctor.

16

Back to the Thalidomide issue.

When the wound stopped ripping, I eventually was put on other wound treatment with foam to absorb drainage. In late November 2020, I saw a wound care nurse who used silver to cauterize the wound. The drainage cut by half in just that hour.

Shortly after that silver treatment, the gastroenterologist called me and told me, see, it was the Thalidomide that had stopped me from healing. I confronted him about that. It was the silver treatment that promoted the scaring, with results in the same hour, and quite a while had passed since I had been taken off of the Thalidomide, with no effect on healing until the very moment the silver treatment was done. He couldn't argue about it, since these were things that were on record, including the tearing of the wound. Facts on record didn't stop him before, and that didn't stop him now. He waited a short time after that conversation, since he had to come up with a new lie.

He came up with a new lie. He changed his story from Thalidomide preventing healing to Thalidomide being the reason that my colon perforated, and he said that if I ever had Thalidomide again I would lose the rest of my intestines! That was in denial of what happened and contradicted the opinion of the surgeon and ignores the dehydration and impacted colon which the gastroenterologist wouldn't do anything about, and was indirect contradiction of what he himself had said. He had set me up to lose my colon. It also contradicted himself, since he allowed me to remain on Thalidomide for a time after the surgery, which he wouldn't have done if he honestly thought what he was claiming now. Or, there is certainly enough evidence that he was trying to hurt me intentionally, and none of this mess would have happened if it wasn't for his malpractice. He was refusing to ever put me back on the only effective medication. And, of course was still yelling at me about the complaint 5 months after! He pulled my off of my medication in clear retaliation for the complaint.

For the high output, he tried giving me a powder to help bile absorption, which had nothing to do with water absorption, and there had been no indication that I was having a bile problem. I went on the max dose with no effect. Of course, the doctor then prescribed the exact same thing under a different name, like I would be too stupid to notice. There was no effect on the water absorption since that powder doesn't treat active inflammation. The medication that does treat Crohn's Disease was still denied, with the continuation of the "I don't know why you are not feeling well," as well as the direct denials that there is any problem, going so far as to say it is all in my head since the stuff for absorbing bile didn't change my water absorption! It would have been common sense for anyone else to realize that I didn't have a problem absorbing bile and that is why there was no effect. It is something that can be tested for also, but he wasn't about to do a test that would have shown him to be wrong.

17

It wasn't enough to just have that toad living in my stomach, the narcissist wasn't satisfied until the small dwarf was shoved in also.

So, what was it like trying to function with this problem which was created for me? After all, everyone told me how much better my life was going to be without a major organ which was not the problem, and how great life was going to be now that I still had to deal with the Crohn's problem but crippled in new ways that never had to happen.

Eventually, I had to go back to work. We all knew that. I planned for it. I did exercises to get stronger in the ways I needed to function in life and on a construction site. I went back to work in early 2021, which was before the continuous collapse of my health from being pulled off of medication crossed the line where I wouldn't be able to survive.

I was able to absorb some fluid, but not enough to meet my needs, so I couldn't be exposed to heat or sweat much. Luckily, it was winter still. I quickly learned that things got dangerous around 90 degrees, and deadly around 95 degrees. I learned that sweat had to be rationed, and even a matter of minutes of sweating would cause a week of cramps. That meant that there were some jobs I had to refuse, due to the temperature of the location or a combination of that and the activity. Sweating for any reason had to be avoided.

Fluid absorption was variable still, with the absorption ranging from 0% for several days a month to 50% for three days when I would get the otherwise worthless Stelara. 20% absorption was more normal at this point. I was still able to use the three days of 50% absorption to a small advantage, since that was enough to get me through times when I would anticipate a greater danger of dehydration, and I would time the injections accordingly. Three days doesn't get far.

One thing I was able to figure out was that once fluid passed a certain point in my intestine there would be no more absorption of the fluid. To get around that problem and at least get something I had to be taking in fluids as much as possible to keep the functioning intestine continuously wet. I was able to get enough to survive but not be well.

That came with another problem. If fluid doesn't absorb, then obviously it has to go somewhere. That somewhere was into my bag, which allowed me a good indication of the amount of absorption most of the time, and the amount going into the bag could be compared to the amount going into my bladder. Sometimes that comparison wouldn't work. Sometimes I would go through a gallon of water during the day before noticing that nothing was coming out my bladder or my bag. If nothing was going into my bladder, then eventually at some point it would all come pouring out into my bag. That gallon could come out within the space of an hour later that evening, with a bag that is only a fraction of that volume. It was unfortunate that I couldn't reduce my fluid intake or I wouldn't absorb even the small amount that I do.

Output was very debilitating. At times, the bag would have to be emptied every 10-15 minutes for a few hours straight. It is very difficult to function in any capacity during that time, and that time can happen at any time. It couldn't really be planned for. Even at the other times, with emptying my bag 20-30 times a day, all times are bad, but some times worse than others.

That meant that even if my job only required me to be present at a site, with no physical activity, there was still the problem of just getting to that site. Construction projects don't come to me. I have to go to them, and that could mean driving 1 ½ hours to a typical site in whatever city, going up to 5 hours in one direction for further projects. Getting to a job meant that I also had to get back from that job. Output is always somewhat worse later in the day and at night, which meant that the drive home was worse than the drive to the job site. I had to be ready to deal with my bag at any moment, and sometimes numerous times during the drive to or from. Since my bag would suddenly fill at any moment, that would lead to the extreme situation of having to let my bag drain while stuck in a lane of traffic on the freeway when traffic wasn't moving and I couldn't get to the shoulder or an exit.

Often, I only had less than a minute to deal with the bag when it would suddenly fill. It happened often enough that I would be driving, and so my bag would blow apart before I could do anything. Sometimes the bag would break apart while on a job. I thought about quitting every day. With the bad bags I was trying to deal with early on, I was lucky to get one day before there was a problem with the bag, and sometimes found myself wrapping myself in Gorilla Tape trying to keep the bag in place long enough to get home. Those early bags also had a nasty habit of spontaneously developing holes in the bag while on a job, leaving me trying to patch it somehow. Sometimes bags would just fall off. Being exposed to air temperatures above 90 degrees weakened the adhesive, besides the dehydration danger. I would have to be very careful how I move, and had to learn different ways of performing tasks.

Sometimes a job would require me to stay at a motel. I kept my supplies with me and dealt with changing the bag at the motel. The early bags I could only get maybe a day out of before it wouldn't seal anymore. So, changing bags was very frequent, and would get very painful. I kept supplies for changing bags with me at all times when the supplies would not be exposed to too much heat, since heat made it so the stuff wouldn't even stick for a minute. I kept a change of clothes with me at all times, along with sheets that I could use to make a privacy tent out of my truck to change in.

One of the projects I hated the most was the 6th Street Bridge in Los Angeles. Every time I would go there should have been the last, but I kept being sent there. The activity was not very physical, and the sampling of post-tensioned cable grout didn't involve much. It would have been an easy job, except that sampling of that cable grout would be every 10-20 minutes or so. It was normal that my highest output time (every 10-15 minutes) would happen while I was on that job. My bags kept breaking, and it was very difficult to function. I hated being there, but I couldn't tell anyone there why I was struggling so hard with something that should have been so simple.

One project was at a prison in San Luis Obispo. It would have been a great job, except that driving there and back could take 11 hours on top of the time on site (and I wasn't paid for drive time). Most times there would be work on multiple days and I could stay there, but it was unpredictable and sometimes I would get there and have to go home the same day. The job itself was pleasant, and I wasn't working inside the prison itself but out in the hills with the cows and turkeys. On site it was a rather low stress job, with things proceeding slowly. But a 19 hour day was intolerable, when most of that would be without being right next to a restroom. This was during the Pandemic, when gas stations and so forth closed their restrooms, and I didn't have any time to guess which one was open. I developed a routine for emptying my bag on the road, with supplies handy, and I could dispose of the trash bags when I got where I was going. On a job site, I could be near a restroom most of the time. I worked in construction long enough to know to bring my own toilet paper or paper towels when I went to a restroom so I could clean the bag. Toilet paper often disappears overnight, and it isn't just random homeless people. Construction workers will also clean out the toilet paper before leaving the site. At 3 in the morning it isn't usually possible to find some 24 hour store with a restroom at whatever random location I needed it to be. Every time I had to deal with the bag meant it took that much longer to get somewhere. Driving time could increase an incredible amount for long drives.

That San Luis Obispo job also had me consider quitting every day. There were three reasons I was on that job. One was because out of 140 inspectors at my company for some reason there weren't very many who could pass a background check. One reason was that out of the tiny pool of people who could pass a background check almost all refused to drive that far. The third reason I was there was because it is so close to the ocean that the temperature stayed in my range when it was too hot in most of Southern California. The town was a nice, calm town and there was a park I could go to and swing. I went for short walks. I found that walking around a town is necessary. I couldn't stay away from a restroom very long, especially later in the day. My walks stayed short, with many very close calls. After a certain number of times showing up there and finding out that I would have to go back home, I had to stop going to that one. The strain was too much and was having an impact on my health, which was bad enough.

During that time, things were getting worse, with my diet becoming more and more restricted as more and more foods would fail to break down. I had to rely more and more on milk. I'm used to that after so many years, so that wasn't a problem. I just adjusted as things became uneatable. Most of those foods were not really missed, though, since they were still plants at this stage and I couldn't get any nutrition out of them anyway. It's just hard to go without plants in this society. Plants are mixed into everything.

It was also during the time at San Luis Obispo that I switched to a better brand of ostomy supplies. I found a cheap bag out of China for a dollar a bag that was far superior to the high end $10 per bag stuff. I combined it with a paste called Stomahesive. With this combination I could get 5 days between bag changes. Also, the cheap bags never developed random holes in the plastic. I had been desperate enough to try to bond the bags using silicone adhesive, which is the only reason I could get even one day out of the other bags and make it through a day of work most of the time. I searched online, reading reviews for bags. I found a cheap brand where I found some bad ratings. Reading the ratings, it sounded exactly like what I needed. Someone with a normal case had given a bad rating because it bonded so well that it ripped the skin when being changed! It doesn't bond anywhere close to that degree with me, but it was exactly what I needed and allowed me to function better. It was only a problem every five days. Changing a bag is anywhere from stressful to borderline traumatic. It is a tricky process, with output coming out while trying to change the bag. I would have to shut off my digestive tract during that time with the tincture of opium, or it would be nearly impossible with stool spraying and no bag on. Then, I have to try not to move for 6 hours after changing the bag or the seal would be broken and the process would have to be started all over. Sometimes I would have to do that several times during a day and night because something went wrong and it didn't seal. I couldn't sleep during that 6 hours because I could accidentally move wrong and break the seal before it set. It would be very difficult to go to a job after a night of that. It would be when the bag would have to be changed multiple times within a day that my skin would get ripped. Changing the bag was a very big deal. Most of the time that wouldn't happen and I would get the full five days.

It was also during the time at San Luis Obispo that things went even further with the people at the church. They were stalking us as bad as what the media says about Scientologists during that time, with them even being brazen enough to pull into my driveway at night right after I got home and snap pictures right there in my driveway. They took off when I stepped out of the house. They were taking pictures of my truck, which was now home. They came back in a matter of minutes, and I went out. They had gotten the info they wanted when they saw I was home. We kept that white car in memory. Being stalked by members of that church was nothing new, in San Bernardino as well as in Ridgecrest, where professional stalkers were even hired to follow me and terrorize me, and members of the church in Ridgecrest even admitted involvement. The private investigator they sent after me was only one of them, and the least threatening of the mercenaries they hired. The San Bernardino ones went further than just spying on me and my house, and I will describe below what they tried to do with Amy. It was devastating to find this out while I was in the motel room. Amy knew never to tell anyone when I was out of town. They were still trying to use my time of weakness to destroy us. This only showed the extent of the betrayal, which we were unaware of at the time, although there were signs. At least they saw me standing, walking and obviously not as vulnerable as they hoped. That would help, but we had to be ready to protect ourselves at all times. It wasn't an isolated incident, and so the campaign of terror against us continued. We had to watch at all times. I don't know any line these people won't cross. They kept watching us. Our neighbor had just before that set up a tall wood fence in their yard, which made it so our house couldn't be watched from down the street. Hence, they had to drive up to our house in the cul-de-sac as they did. That was helpful. It also meant that it was more important to be home where I could protect us, even if it was just by deterrence of my presence. Traveling overnight still would happen.

During the summer it was necessary to turn down jobs in hot areas. I stayed by the coast when possible. Sometimes it was possible to do a job in my area if it was only in the morning and I could get out of there before the temperature hit the magic number when everything in my life falls apart, literally. Once, they insisted that I go to El Centro, because I was the only person who could do that particular activity. I had to refuse, and after a number of days had to threaten to quit if they tried to send me. I can't handle that heat for even a minute.

There were other jobs that were remodels of existing buildings. That was usually a good option because those buildings usually had air conditioning. Many of those jobs were at night. One job was during the day and was on a roof, with temperatures going over 100 degrees on the roof. The roof had an air conditioned mechanical penthouse where I could stay out of the heat, coming out only for a few minutes at a time when I needed to look at something, back in the penthouse before the sweating would set in. Another job, which was enjoyable in a way, was testing welds on a 30' diameter water main that was around 15 feet below a road. I would crawl from manhole to manhole, with about a quarter of a mile of pipe that I crawled through. It was

100 degrees up on the surface but below 70 degrees in the pipe. The only problem was having to crawl fast enough to get to the surface to empty my bag at the most inconvenient moments.

There were adjustments to make regarding scheduling eating or drinking. I had to learn the time it takes things to go through me. Most of the liquids would go through me in the range of 4-8 hours, with some later. Most of the solid food would go through in the 8-20 hour range, with some lasting up to two days. That meant that there was sometimes a pattern to the output, although it was only some of the time with the rest of the days being unpredictable. To help with sleeping, it was necessary to stop eating solid food by 11:00AM. That meant that enough of the stuff would be out by 9:00PM so I could get a few hours of sleep. Otherwise, the output may be every half hour all night, which would still happen every few days anyway no matter what I did. Even if I had to empty the bag every hour, that meant not sleeping at all. Once I could get to sleep there would be a small reduction in output, but I have to get to sleep first to get that small improvement. That resulted in the conundrum that the output had to slow in order to slow the output. Chicken or the egg? They both taste good with enough salt and pepper.

It was important to have low output at the times I would have to spend driving for however long. Early morning was usually a higher output time, except that when I would spend the entire night emptying my bag there was usually very little output by the time I needed to be somewhere. The output also had to stop long enough for me to leave the house. Later in the afternoon was when the output from whatever I drank early in the morning would increase, getting more difficult as it got later. If I was lucky it would peak after I got home. Then, after home, it was better to get as much out as fast as possible. It was not possible solve the problem. It all has to come out at some time. The trick was to adjust the time to sometime more convenient, when the least would be sacrificed.

18

Back in late 2020, narcissists smelled blood. Besides the stuff Amy's family was doing to harm us, things got worse with certain members of the church.

I had only just recovered enough to continue my ecclesiastical duties to some degree. I hadn't gained much strength, but was getting stronger. One Sunday in December, I taught the other priests again for the first time since the surgery. That exposed weakness, and they could all see the weakness even on Zoom over a computer screen, since this was in the Pandemic. I hadn't slept before, which was not unusual. None of those cowards would have done what they did if they thought I could resist. They didn't think I could resist in my condition.

Like in July, I got a call from the guy who had assigned the lesson to me. He noted my condition, and then proceeded to try to tear me apart. He gave me some familiar orders, which reminded me of a company I had been with a while back as discussed above. I was ordered to not quote anything, not even the assigned speech from the conference which I had been assigned to discuss. I was to read the title of the speech, and that was it. In every discussion, this leader would try to make each lesson his personal forum, generally preventing discussion as much as possible. It was very difficult to get through a lesson with him hijacking the discussion. I had given the discussions exactly on the subject of the speeches assigned. He asked if I even pray. Yes I do. I pray about each lesson for at least two weeks, going over and over the assigned speeches until I understood each aspect of the message. He told me that I am the reason that no one can feel the Spirit. Like all narcissists, he claimed that "the brethren" were the ones who had complained about me and that this stuff he was saying was supposedly coming from them not him. That was in direct contradiction to what the others had told me themselves, including feeling the Spirit. One thing that is a basic fact about narcissists is that 90% of the time they are flat out lying about the conversations they claim to have had with others about you. This was one of those cases, but that doesn't mean that the others were not involved, or that they were safe people.

He proceeded to accuse me of an "agenda". How? He was the one who decided what was to be taught. Other awful stuff was said about me. He told me that my knowledge was "intellectualism". Typical of narcissists to deny anything deep. I got my knowledge from the brink of death. I put in the work to know the meaning of things. I can't even share much of it with them since they would have to experience it themselves. People have demanded that I share things I can't share, and when I couldn't do that (since it doesn't work like that) they tried to take it away from me. This group of people were no different, and I was known to be an expert in certain things. He asked me "Do you even want this calling?" in a very hostile and sarcastic tone. I responded " It isn't about wanting or not wanting this calling!" He gasped. He ended the conversation very quickly after that. Narcissists can't handle someone who speaks up. He also knows that I was right about it and there was nothing he could say in response which would not expose him as a power freak. There was also much more he said. He was still in a rage from July also when I stood up to him then and referenced that incident.

The following week I tried to share something deeply personal, and had my testimony openly mocked by the WHOLE group.

I hadn't mentioned to Amy what was happening or what had happened back in July. It is important to note that the cowards didn't pull this stuff when I was doing well. They only made their moves at a moment of apparent weakness.

Shortly after the December incident, when they all mocked me in the meeting, Amy told me of a dream she just had. In the dream she saw a conspiracy among the members of the church, and they were seeking our destruction. They were in real life. I then told her how I was being treated.

The men had been quite nice, with some exceptions, up till then. The women in the church were mostly very hostile and outright dangerous. The men had always been more of a refuge, which even the women commonly admitted. It was very common for the women who are excluded from the clique to find the refuge among the men that was denied to them by the women, who have their own group. That group of women kick out people with differences, telling them that they don't belong there. Very few of the marginalized women stay, and actually I can only think of one, and she only stayed by avoiding the women as much as possible and staying closer to the men, who she told me didn't treat her so awful, with one exception. She pointed to that guy while yelling "Except for him!" Still, it was a story I had heard from women all my life, and many women join the church but very few stay more than a few months. All the while, the women *demand* praise while destroying everyone they can.

My cat reminds me of an important fact in nature. It is to be found in all of nature, including humans. My cat has extra toes. The litter was born on top of our patio cover. This kitten was different, not fitting what a kitten is *supposed* to be, so the mother decided to kill him, which is normal in the animal world. It is common in the human world too, and killing anyone different seems to be the one real maternal instinct. I have met many human mothers who are not that way, and according to the media it isn't like that in general society, but that was not my experience. Not everyone is that lucky, and I got a narcissistic cat mother, and I was supposed to die for being different. I have found the women in this church to be that way. There were lines that the men in the church have NEVER crossed, but I know no line that the women in this church won't cross and have. It wasn't the men giving me death threats. It also wasn't the men who were claiming that our son was kidnapped by us and isn't our son. Very few men, but what seemed to be most of the women, claimed that I have no faith or I would have been healed long ago, and only the women in the church have claimed that my illness is proof of how evil I am and I am being punished by God. I can't remember any of the men saying that. At the same time, men who will stand up for us are very few to none, so I can't respect them for being afraid to do what is right.

Amy and I decided that we needed to take these matters up the chain. We met with a higher leader about it. We told him all that happened. It is notable that as we arrived for the meeting at the church another person of the group of priests said "How's my favorite teacher?" He was one of the "brethren" who the other guy told me was complaining about me. I already knew the narcissist was lying about it since I grew up around narcissists and I'm used to hearing about conversations which are proven to have never happened. That is why they often won't give names, so you can't go and ask that person if they really said what was claimed. After praying about the situation, Amy and I had come to the conclusion that we needed to attend a church in another area, due to the danger to us. The hatred toward us had reached the point where if we went to the church we would have to go armed. I didn't want to do that, but only out of respect toward God and not because I have any problem protecting myself or Amy and Quinn. It was best that we attend elsewhere. There was also a series of email that with him that I still have as proof of what was discussed and what I reported as going on. It is proof that he was told. We explained that we are not leaving the religion. We are just trying to protect ourselves.

That leader found our solution to be reasonable, and he expressed support. We found another group to attend in Fontana. It had to be far enough away. That leader also approved of us taking the matter to a higher level. I felt that was necessary due to the nature of what was going on.

The meeting with the even higher leader went pretty much the same way.

It was now 2021. What we didn't know at the time was that leader we had the first meeting with called ahead to that group in Fontana and made sure that we would not be accepted there. It worked. They did not accept us. They tried to discourage us from attending, and told me that I can't hold any position in that group. I was not seeking any position. We were only seeking to practice our religion in peace and safety. I don't care about ranks and titles. The Sneetches who drove us to this point were obsessed with getting stars on their bellies, and projection is a weapon they use.

I should have known that we would be betrayed, and I had hoped that it was just a misunderstanding. In the later Spring in 2021, I was in San Luis Obispo. Amy had a meeting with that leader who we had the first meeting with. When he had her alone, everything changed. The he tried to convince her that she really wants to be back in that group and somehow I am stopping her. That was a conscious lie, since Amy had told him of her dream in in the earlier meeting and he knew it wasn't me controlling her and stopping her from coming. He knew that SHE had warned me of the danger. It was explained to him completely by HER, not by me, so there is no excuse. He also claimed that I don't give any donations because I wasn't putting money directly into his hands. He knew that I made donations online like the majority of the people do when they give a donation. We hadn't been meeting in person during the Pandemic, online donations were considered normal and that was the best method. When Amy said that I do make donations online, he tried to convince her that I don't, asking her how she would know. It is really simple. I just pull up my account on the website and show the donation record to prove it, but this was not about facts which he already knew. In order to convince her to attend that group, he dangled a position for her. But even that turned into an attack on me. He said "We *know* what Ethan thinks about callings, but what do you think?" Amy wasn't tricked by this. One of the emails I had sent that guy had said that I can't fill my position with the narcissistic abuse I was going through. Nowhere does that say that I have a problem with filling a position. I have the email as proof, but this is a liar we were dealing with. Lying has nothing to do with known facts.

So, with the extent of the betrayal clear, we needed a new plan. There are local groups with usually several in a city. There is a larger grouping of several of those groups. We would have to go outside of that larger group to a different region, since we had also betrayed by the leader of that larger group. We would not tell anyone where we were going, or they would try to drive us out of that group. It had to be far enough away so the spy network would have a more difficult time tracking us. Also, it was better to let them think that we had left the religion, which they had already been claiming (there was a bunch of stuff said to Amy). If they thought they had finally driven us out of the religion, they could use that as proof of our deserving murderous hatred, and they might not look for us. This bought us a long time, but narcissists never let a victim go. More on that later.

The group we went to accepted us. Things were very different. The women were also very different. Even the women in this group took the religion seriously and took an active part in discussions, which I had never seen before in my life. I have never seen such a thing in this religion in my entire life until now. The leader of the women, who is a woman, was not a narcissist. That was a first for me also. There were no cliques I could see in this group. There was a level of respect among this group I have never seen in my life anywhere, not just in this religion. This group actually *wanted* us to be there. They considered us to be one of them. This was how everything is supposed to be. These were people I could call Christian because they were actually following it rather than just saying it. They cared about us, and were concerned about how we were doing. They knew we were having serious trouble in every way, but they did not cross any boundaries and they followed the policy of the church to respect us and our autonomy. But they let us knew that they were ready to help if we needed it. No coercion. No violation of individual sovereignty. No one trying to take over our lives. No one telling us how we deserve to be hated. No one telling us we are going to burn in hell for having problems. They were safe. They were safe like I never thought possible among a group of people. Just like I learned about Baptists long ago when I left Ridgecrest, it stands to reason that there are more people out there who take their religion seriously. I just found the bad ones first before finding the good ones. It points out that there are good and bad in all religious groups and all other divisions of society outside of religion. The problem is that the bad ones are the ones who are most active and most vocal and suck up all the attention like vampires. The good ones are the ones who leave people alone, so they don't get much publicity. Cedars-Sinai is also one of those exceptions I had come across. I found Cedars-Sinai after and among the bad experiences. If all I knew was Kaiser or Loma Linda I would have no hope to continue surviving. I would have no faith in the medical profession if they were all I knew. I would have a deep hatred of all nurses if I hadn't found them all different at Cedars-Sinai. The ones at Kaiser and Loma Linda did a real good job of demonstrating that compassion and caring are not a natural instinct. Cedars-Sinai showed me that it might be if people want it to be. Loma Linda showed me the worst that supposedly Christian care can become, and what happens if you are not part of their clique. Cedars-Sinai showed me that a hospital associated with a particular religion can be very respectful and care about everyone, even having a service to arrange any religious services for anyone of any religion without hatred and withholding care. They may not have been rated the top in the world, but they cared, and for me and my set of issues that placed them at the top of what I needed, and they were the ones who recognized that a disease is not just physical, but social and spiritual and so forth. They are concerned about all aspects of the problem. The new church group I was with was the wonderful exception to my experiences. We found peace and a place of safety, for now. I don't want to sound biased toward certain groups, but my experiences have been particularly bad with few exceptions. I can't deny what happened, even if saying it is not in line with the popular view of how things are "supposed" to be. Even though I keep bringing up certain demographics it is because certain ones have been more extreme in their hatred and actions toward us, but the problem is among all divisions of society, among all people, and the problem is not limited to one gender or religion or profession. Some people have crossed lines that others didn't. Some groups crossed other lines. But one thing is certain, that things are NOT the way they are *supposed* to be. There is a toxic masculinity too, and I run into that all the time in my job, particularly when people notice that I'm not as tall as other people. But toxic masculinity is also not limited to men, even though certain people in the church insist that only men are evil and women are all naturally born good and are automatically good no matter what they do to destroy people, while I have been informed that I am automatically damned to hell because of my gender. (There is actually a long list of other reasons why people have said I am damned automatically, yet all of those reasons have been stated by women. Men have never told me I am damned, even the ones who hate me have never said that. I have been hearing it from women all my life.) Maybe someone else has experienced things that match certain ideals, but that has not been my experience as a general trend. If people want me to think otherwise then they are going to have to stop proving my experiences to be an accurate representation of things. Some people have done a good job of proving my experiences to be the exception, but the bad outweighs the good by a large proportion.

I have known many women who have experienced the same thing in reverse that I went through, and just as bad. I read the stories of countless other women in articles. Sometimes it is the father who is the narcissist rather than having a very dangerous narcissist mother and a completely passive father like I had. They are justified in making the corresponding conclusions that their life experiences have shown them to be fact.

I have been hurt and betrayed by countless men also.

The point is that no one is automatically born good and automatically worthy of being "saved" while another group (gender, ethnicity, religion, etc.) is automatically evil and damned. Such things are the foundation of aristocracy, which is at the root of many evils. Think of how evil was associated with "commoners" to the point that certain words reinforcing the automatically good aristocrat and automatically evil commoner have remained to this day. People still speak of "villains" who live in the village rather than the lord's manor. Someone who causes harm is called "mean", which literally means average or common. Look how the aristocrats are still called "our betters". Yet it is the lords who gave us the word "entitled". The "nobles", meaning they don't mix and are separate from all those without stars on their bellies, have been the ones in every society who are robbers, rapists, murderers, the greediest, and hide behind their supposedly God given privilege as an excuse why they are automatically good no matter what they do, while all their victims are damned for being born in less privileged circumstances. "Noble" means predator above all other meanings, and no claims of divine right changes that fact.

When a particular group of women drive out any woman different than them, and all you have are the narcissists left since narcissists back up other narcissists and don't find anything wrong with *them,* then all you get to see is the clique. The normal women who are good people disappear really fast and are therefore not represented by this group. It doesn't help that this was the case in every church group I went to until this very last one. At Kaiser and Loma Linda, they seem to seek out the particularly awful women to be nurses, and the most narcissistic of the women to be doctors. That is what happens any time there is a narcissist in charge. Narcissists need validation for all the evil they do, so they are comfortable around people just like them since if "everyone" does it like they insist, then they can pretend that their actions aren't as bad or exceptional as they really are. The men in this church have been very different than the women in every group I have been with, and have been much more inclusive and accepting of people with differences, including people with severe mental illnesses, who had been rejected by the women. The acceptance, of course, didn't apply to me.

These new people helped giving me hope for human beings. I didn't hear them talk trash about certain other members of society the way all other groups I had been with had. It is a violation of church rules to be doing that, but rules are not enforced, so trash talk of marginalized groups in society often happens. But, it must be remembered that they are doing that in violation of the rules, not because of the rules or because of the actual position of the church on various matters. Contrary to what certain individuals want the world to think, this is not an authoritarian religion. People can think believe what they want, and they can say so and do, especially when they forget to take their medication. The problem with the "honor system" is that it requires honor.

In December, 2021, I was back at the 6th St bridge in Los Angeles. I began having symptoms of my intestines shutting down, with vomiting. I had barely been able to tolerate even liquids. I called the dispatcher and they were able to find someone who could replace me. I stayed for a couple hours to help get the harder part of the work out of the way, and then went home and to the hospital. What happened at the hospital was important information, even if it wasn't new information. My gastroenterologist stayed out of it like usual. I was given solumedrol, which is an intravenous steroid, which I had been given the summer before. By the next day I was symptom free, like the summer before. The important point was that my problem was completely treatable since it was active inflammation. I was released a few days later, but they didn't give me anything to keep the inflammation under control and just sent me home unmedicated. Solumedrol is fast acting, but short acting. I was back in the hospital in a number of days. This time they kept giving me the solumedrol during the whole stay, and it knocked down the inflammation enough to have me stable for some time. It cured the dull constant pain that I had ever since doing the prep for the colonoscopy.

In December 2021, the gastroenterologist brought up a double-balloon enteroscopy. He asked if I was willing to do it. There was only one Kaiser around where it is done. I said I would do it. This was the one chance to get him to admit to the active disease, since no other scope is able to reach the bad areas from either direction. He said he would write the order. Nothing happened. When I talked to him next, he said he didn't write the order because I refused to say I would do it! I repeated again that I would do it if he would give the order. He then said "Would you *REALLY* do it?!" I said yes, but he just kept repeating that accusatory question. He wouldn't write the order, and this kept happening over a number of months. One idea which had been brought up was getting a referral back to the IBD Center at Cedars-Sinai. They have always been able to fix the damage Kaiser has done to ne every time, so since my gastroenterologist was refusing to allow the one test that would prove me right, I asked for a referral to Cedars-Sinai, which he gave.

During this time, he had continued the gaslighting, with the claims that my Crohn's problem is literally in my head. Rather than prescribe the medication which would help me, he prescribed an anti-depressant! I didn't refuse, since I am not going to refuse a sleeping pill, no matter how little it does. It would take Michael Jackson's doctor to really treat my insomnia. It may have killed him, but it worked.

I was able to get a referral to Cedars-Sinai in 2022. I went there, with only one visit being approved. I discussed the situation, and recommendations were given. It was also suggested that I find a new gastroenterologist at Kaiser. There was a gastroenterologist at the Kaiser in Baldwin Park, which is where the double-balloon enteroscopy is performed. So, I went to that person.

That person was even worse than the first. I had more than one visit, and things went pretty bad, with this doctor crossing even more lines. She insisted now, without testing, that I have short bowel syndrome, which is something proven that I don't have since I haven't lost enough intestine to cause that. She said I am not absorbing anything, declared me to have low protein from malnutrition, even though the blood test showed that my protein levels were actually higher than the normal range, showing that my diet was working just fine and I was still absorbing animal protein as I had already explained. Next she talked about my vitamin D problem, which I do have a problem with. She said I need to take 50000 units a week for a short time. That had never worked. I had been on 50000 units each day for a long time to get the levels in range. My endocrinologist even had me taking 100000 units a day for a time. The idea was that if the parathyroid tumor was removed and and my vitamin D levels were not extra high then hungry-bone syndrome might happen. The endocrinologist had been telling me over the phone to take those doses without writing a prescription, since it is over the counter. The gastroenterologist then argued that 50000 unit capsules don't exist over the counter! So much for Kaiser and elementary school math. I never said it was one capsule, since I can count. I had to explain to this "doctor" than they come in 5000 unit capsules over the counter and 10x5=50! They now come in 10000 unit capsules. She then snapped "That's too much!" It is too much or am I still malnourished? Which one is it. She was just shifting her story to oppose me like a toddler. She also looked at the blood results and said that my vitamin D levels were too high, which they were do to preparing for the possible parathyroid surgery, but then still insisted that I don't absorb it. If I can't absorb it, then taking more of it won't hurt anything. She both wanted me to stop taking vitamin D and insisted that I can't absorb it. She insisted that the only reason that I don't absorb some things is because my bowel is so short it just shoots through me like a laser beam. It is on record how much intestine I have lost, and therefore how much intestine I still have. When I explained how long it actually takes for food to go through (one to two days) she snapped "That doesn't count!" She did do a 72 hour stool fat count. When the results showed that I was absorbing fats, although below average, she wrote that I have NO absorption of ANYTHIG in the notes. She also declared my case untreatable.

Of the everything she refused to listen to, she saw the hole in my abdomen and automatically declared it to be a fistula. She wouldn't give me any medication unless it is proven that it is not a fistula. I had explained what had happed after the surgery and that it is on record with countless photos showing the ripped suture. I don't have a fistulizing type of Crohn's. She ignored me.

She referred me to a surgeon. I went to see the surgeon, since that would be the only way to get her to give me the medication I need to survive, and survival was getting very difficult. I was starting to have tremors and getting shaky, with the pain coming back quite strong. The tremors were related to the pain. It was getting hard to function.

I saw the surgeon in the fall of 2022. He walked into the room and said "You don't have a fistula." He recognized the hole as a suture hole, and said he sees it all the time. He said he would call the doctor immediately to tell her that I am not a candidate for surgery and she needs to put me back on Thalidomide immediately. Another surgery would destroy my life and possibly *cause* short bowel syndrome. He also didn't think I had a good chance of surviving the surgery in the condition Kaiser had put me in.

She had also had me taking enzymes. I had told her that enzymes had been tried in the past, but she insisted that this was different, without finding out what enzymes had already been tried. Also, testing for enzymes did not show me to have any deficiency of enzymes. That should have also been obvious since I wasn't having a problem absorbing enough of the things like proteins and fats from my diet without extra enzymes. Things got noticeably worse with the enzymes. I had warned her that it was making things worse, with my water absorption even dropping by half of what it had been, and she insisted that I keep taking the stuff which was making it impossible for me to survive. I stopped the enzymes and my water absorption returned to what it had been, which was just enough to survive under the right conditions. She also wouldn't order the double balloon enteroscopy.

So I waited a while. Eventually, the gastroenterologist, instead of getting me the medication I need, which even the surgeon told her I need, referred me to another surgeon! It was obvious that I was dealing with an even worse narcissist than before, and she had no regard for my life. It was very conclusive that I was not being treated in good faith, and her intention was to hurt me. I was not being treated in good faith, and the retaliation against me was continuing. I was being punished by Kaiser for the complaint, still. She didn't like the answer the surgeon gave, since it showed her to be wrong, so she was doing the typical narcissist thing of hunting around for someone who will say what she wants to hear, just like my mother did to try to stop my son from being treated. I saw that they would kill me if I stayed at Kaiser. Narcissists always back eachother up against the victims, and she was continuing the abuse from the first one, except taking it to a level the first one wouldn't go. The surgeon had told me that she treats things aggressively, but obviously that didn't apply to *me.* None of the recommendations from the doctor at Cedars-Sinai were following. All of those recommendations were ignored.

I requested a referral to another doctor, but she tried to block that. She was offended that I wanted another opinion before throwing away my life to please her ego. She said that she has no power to give referrals, even though she had been making referrals. More lies from Kaiser directed toward stopping me from getting help. I was able to get a referral from another doctor, and I set up an appointment with a gastroenterologist. Knowing that narcissists don't let go of any victim, and knowing that the abuse by proxy would continue with a new doctor, I didn't keep that appointment, since the gastroenterologist would have been watching my record to see the referral she didn't want me to have and would contact that new doctor to prevent me from getting help. I had to change insurance before Kaiser kills me. My only chance of surviving would be to get back to Cedars-Sinai. I would have to do it fast because of my deteriorating condition.

In December 2022 I was able to work it out with the union to get a different insurance that would allow me to get to Cedars-Sinai. It would take months to actually get in. In that time, things kept getting worse, and eventually eating or drinking anything was becoming a problem, with actual malnutrition beginning to set in. When I finally did get to Cedars-Sinai, I had to face all the lies and bogus reports the Kaiser doctors had placed on my record to stop me from getting help anywhere I try to go. They knew that any doctor would not have time to actually look at the test results and would just go by the brief summary that those liars made up in opposition to the actual test results. It would be a long process, and it was hard to get listened to after what Kaiser did to me.

Among the things they wrote was that there is NO inflammation going on and that NO test showed any sign of inflammation, which was a lie since it had shown up just fine in the scan in 2020 before the steroids and also the calprotectin levels of 650 plus and high C-reactive protein levels and sedimentation rate. They had written that I have NO ABOSRPTION OF ANYTHING. How am I alive then, since I hadn't lost any more small intestine since 1997. They declared, without any testing that I have short bowel syndrome, yet it had been declared by both surgeons and doctors that I could lose more intestine before reaching that point, and besides, I asked one doctor, if I had short bowel syndrome then how did I survive all these years just fine on my diet when I hadn't had any TPN since the beginning of the 1990s? He thought that was a good point, which it is. The Kaiser doctors were making these declarations to stop anyone from helping me, and had declared me untreatable with medication. Every time I was given steroids I would go symptom free, so it hardly takes much of a brain to see that there was active disease. But only Cedars-Sinai would prove to have the honesty to do tests and admit what those tests showed, because that is what happened when they did the tests themselves in spite of what Kaiser said. They also wrote that I had chosen to go off of medication! They took me off against my will, and I couldn't even get the mostly worthless Stelara anymore. It would take a while to sort through all the lies Kaiser hurt me with. The Cedars-Sinai gastroenterologist saw that my case was quite complicated and referred me to the IBD Center. It would take some time to get in. He had referred me to the doctor I had seen for quite some time there, but I would be considered a new patient, and he was no longer seeing new patients, so I ended up back with the doctor I had seen that one time in 2022.

Then, on the way to a job, I was having to fight extra hard to get there with output problems. When I did get there, I had lost the strength to get out of the car. I called the dispatcher and Amy to tell them that I had to go to the hospital.

20

Things were not quiet in the religious realm either. During this time in the Fall 2022, the predators smelled blood somehow. They had been trying to track down where we had been attending church. At this point, they changed their tactics and came to our door. They tried to get our son to tell them where we had been going. He didn't. I came to the door to see what was going on. It was the traitor leaders. They told me to come back. I told them that became impossible when things reached the point that I would have to go armed. I confronted them about what they tried to do to Amy when they got her alone. They whispered that they didn't know what I was talking about. I got specific with what they told her. They whispered (knowing Amy was in the living room and they didn't want her to hear what they were saying) denying that it ever happened. I called to Amy "Hey Amy, guess what they say never happened!" Amy came to the door and confronted them about the lies they fed her about me, calling them out on their lies to destroy us. The higher leader who was the one directing the attacks on us then said "I think we should..." I cut him off and said "I think you better get off of my property." They backed away and got out of there. I noticed the particular white car they had…

It is strange how narcissists like them assume that they have been so successful that no one will compare notes. It is strange how they could seek to isolate me like that, try to convince Amy that I am an apostate, and then come to my house like they are my friends. It has been said that narcissists must all read the same manual on how to be narcissists since they all say and do the exact same things, mannerisms, speech patterns and all. They are all very predictable since nothing ever changes. And they all think it will work for some reason.

We were still safe at the place we were going. We had made the correct choice of group, and they hadn't betrayed us to the spy network.

A certain concept should be mentioned at this point. There are countless cases like this, with the exception that I don't know of any other case where someone stayed with the religion. When they flee for their lives they disappear completely from the religion. Things tend to be too close knit, and moving usually won't work to protect someone. Like all groups of society, whether it is religious, business or just social groups, the medical profession, even pedophiles are protected while victims are condemned without forgiveness for being victimized by a predator. There is always the "How dare you accuse them of doing that!" attitude, with all the hatred hell can muster to follow. The people who claim that they don't judge are the most judgmental people of all, since they always judge the victims of crimes and abuse.

But at this point it should be mentioned another side of the matter that I can't condone. That is when even victims will in fact lie to spread hatred in revenge for what happened, and I can't support that. Enough blood has been spilled already.

Some cases are when some woman got caught starting her own cult, and was very hostile to the church, which hostility resulted in her leaving the church. I saw an interview with her afterward, and she made the declaration that the church teaches that a woman must "almost NEVER" work outside the home. That is a lie, and has been from the beginning. If that was true, then why do so many of the women work outside the home and are not just in good standing in the church without being bothered about it, but even hold positions? Even the mayor of San Bernardino a number of years ago (a woman in this church) was in good standing. Statements like that one person said shows an intentional ignorance of what is in plain sight. Even in the beginning the church wanted women to run the businesses, become doctors and lawyers and so forth. This stuff isn't hidden. Not knowing it is serious negligence. There are always some people everywhere who you can find who will deny these facts, but they are not the church and speak only of their own personal views in opposition to the church. They are also predators, since only predators have such extreme gender role stereotypes. We have been warned all my life and long before that you have to be very careful with who you listen to, and everything must be verified. Anything else is a failure.

What people are willing to deny with their eyes open to what is right in front of them all around reminds me of the people who claimed that the color blue would hurt me. They had tried flipping the problem around to new nonsense. They would say it even when I was wearing something blue, and yet they had blinded themselves to it, preferring to only look at the Ethan they made up in their heads. Militant stupidity.

Another case was someone who has also gone through attempted murder and escaped the church in Ridgecrest, with the guy trying to kill her remaining in good standing. She claimed that she had a miscarriage, and was sent by the church to some camp for miscarriages, where they treated her like trash and tore her down. She claimed that it was mandatory in the church. If so, then all women who have miscarriages would be sent there, including Amy. But there is no such thing in the church. One thing that does happen is that there are people who will set up their own personal workshops and classes and teach their own ideas. People have been warned about those, but we have no law against it. That is how murder cults start, and there are many more than the ones which make the news. People have been warned. An unfortunate fact is that those predators target the women specifically, since the women are the least likely to look anything up or question anything told to them. The women are also most likely to believe that this stuff is coming from the church. Anything coming from the church education system can easily be verified through the church website. You can verify anything someone claims is a doctrine of the church, and you can also verify if some workshop is actually being done by the church, because if it is a part of the church then it will be the same workshop everywhere, not just in some isolated spot and nowhere else. It has always been the women, and never once a man in the church, who told me I was being evil for looking and studying things so that I would understand things for myself. But, that is a commandment. Also, Jesus said "Whosoever treasureth up my words shall NOT be deceived." It should be very simple. Besides those people setting up themselves as teachers of secret groups, there are also the books people write. We have no law against people writing books of their own views, but very disturbing things also get published, and people try to say that it is the church that teaches that stuff. Anything from the church is published by the church, since the church is its own publisher. The other stuff people publish are published through a private publisher, which even though it has ties to the church, it is not the church publisher and is still just a private company which will publish any nonsense from anyone. I can't get people to look at the difference, and the fiction writing is the worst of all, since people can't seem to understand that fiction is not real. Just because something can be found in a bookstore that does not imply any endorsement from the church, and people need to be very selective of what they choose to believe, and verify everything. It doesn't matter what position someone may hold in the church organization, if they publish a book it is to state that those are their own opinions and they are responsible for any errors. No one is exempt from that, up to and including the president of the church. If that disclaimer is not there, then the person is in violation of the rules and is suspect. People outside of the church need to be careful what book they claim was published by the church, and what they claim represents official doctrine. People in the church have failed, and they have no one to blame for their negligence but themselves. Those who don't look and know things for themselves are already deceived. When someone (it has always been one of the women) say some ridiculous thing that goes against the actual doctrine or fact, they then tell me "But so-and-so said..." They never bothered to look, and it has messed up their lives immensely by listening to the wrong person. It doesn't matter who that wrong person is. I don't care what their mommy says. It is not against the law of the church for people to believe whatever they want, and the freedom to do so is actually enshrined. No one would be able to joint without the freedom of belief. Otherwise, as it is written, people would be placed on unequal ground due to people not sharing the same experiences or understanding of things. Real knowledge comes from experience, and everyone is in their own place. When someone joins, they need to evaluate what they have. They need to keep everything good that they already have, and learn to replace destructive and self-sabotaging beliefs, as they discover them, with healthier things if they can find them. We are taught to seek that which is virtuous, lovely, of good report or praiseworthy wherever it is, from whatever source. Progress is personal. Most people never give up the unhealthy ideas and interpretations they grew up with.

Spiritual survival is something which must be fought for, like the physical, and it will not bring anyone friends. We have even been warned outright in a world conference that standing up for what is right will mean standing *against* other members of this church. And so it does mean that. I have to be much harder on those of this church, because they have been freely taught these principles, and can't claim ignorance. Other religious groups (most) were not taught such things and are in a different category. I am not talking about the smaller hypocrisies of so many who are only willing to put on an empty show of religion one day a week, whores to society the rest of the time. Hypocrisy can only exist where there are standards and ideals, with the higher the ideals the greater the hypocrisy to be found, since if there are no standards then there are no standards to violate. What they do to destroy people is another matter. It is a person's free choice to hurt themselves and blind themselves, but to destroy others is not something people have a right to do.

Where does one go when it is the leaders who are carrying on the work of destruction? It still appears to be local matters, with the world level leaders kept mostly in ignorance of the lives destroyed. There is still a feeling of betrayal that won't go away, and a feeling of complete abandonment to my fate. What happens is that the highest leaders take the word of the local leaders that everything is fine, when nothing is right. It isn't the job of the highest leaders to be involved in local affairs, but they are the ones selecting the predators to run things locally, and are refusing to see the problems caused. People would rather listen to happy news, like was explained to me by people in my profession, and anything wrong must be hidden so everyone stays happy. I can't respect that. I have covenants that I made which won't allow me to play that game, or I would have blood on my hands like they do. At the same time, God does not work through a secret police or Gestapo, and such a situation can never be allowed to develop. What it takes is people listening to the cries of the victims for once rather than attacking them. Only then can change happen. Only then will the church be able to live up to its principles. When it is no longer a den of thieves, then maybe it can be a sanctuary with healing for the broken souls (so many of which were broken by them.) The aristocratic tendencies of the people must be eliminated, the cliques dissolved, and all people recognized as equal, or it can't be called Christian.

By their own law, they must comply with the requirements to gain forgiveness. By the law they claim to believe and follow, "And he that repenteth not, and confesseth them not, ye shall bring before the church, and do with him as the scripture saith unto you, either by commandment or by revelation. And this shall ye do that God may be glorified –not because ye forgive not, having not compassion, but that ye may be justified in the eyes of the law, that ye may not offend him who is your lawgiver. Verily I say, for this cause shall ye do these things." By the law they themselves profess, we are to hold people accountable for their crimes against others, and forgiveness must come by compliance with the law upon which forgiveness is predicated, which requires complete change and turning away from what is wrong. Anything other than change is continuing the problem, which means that it has nothing to do with getting over the past, but dealing with the present and future which can't be gotten over until it is over and ended. Anything else is a lie, and condoning what is happening. There are other sections even more explicit that I could quote which are quite damning for them.

I don't expect any of them to repent of their evil or change in any way, since it just doesn't work like that with people who have crossed such lines. I know they will never let me go to live my life in peace with any good people I can find, since that is not how predators operate. They destroy whatever they can't have. I know Kaiser won't ever restore what they stole from me either, since having a conscience might hurt profits.

It has been an unfortunate fact of almost all religions in history that they have been both a weapon of the "elite" and a tool of repression, no matter how good the original intentions may have started out. There is no religion which can't be used for evil purposes, since there is nothing that can't be perverted. Look at the so-called Christians who condemn Islam and yet are trying to turn the United States into the Islamic State. Almost none have ever even read the Quran to see what it says, not to mention the Bible to see what that says. One way almost all religions have oppressed people and become a tool of the "elite" is by restricting knowledge to only a certain privileged few, thereby making the rest of the people dependent. Real religion can only be personal. If it is not found as a part of one self it is just empty words and meaningless motions? Then how can it become a reality to them? If it is not a reality, how can it be empowering? Hence, restrictions to only certain few. If it is personal, then only a thief would try to take for themselves exclusively what belongs equally to someone else. At eh same time, people throughout history have failed to hold onto what is theirs, being perfectly happy with this arrangement.

Black Elk said, "The power of a thing or an act is found in understanding the meaning," as quoted in The Sacred Pipe. When we meet together, the intention is not repeating something we have been told, but to share our personal experience of the religion and principles to that we can all learn from our collective experience. We are to share our different views and different perspectives, that all people can find what is good and avoid what is unhealthy. It is only through the different perspectives that we can see beyond our own eyes and our own understanding. There is power there. It only happens sometimes. It happened before certain people took power and made it about enforcing their garbage on others in denial of the religion. They all know that once they crossed that lines they did, misusing their position for narcissistic self-aggrandizement, no one is required to recognize them as having any authority because they violated the ethics and trust of their position, besides the crimes committed. When speaking to people of any religion, I prefer to speak to those who know things for themselves. I have studies many religions, as we have been taught to do. I am less interested in hearing things simply regurgitated, or people simply repeating what they were told to say. That doesn't take any more intelligence than what a bird has, and it doesn't necessarily even have any more personal meaning to them than it would to a cockatoo. I want what is real. Show me the reality of what it means to you. I want to hear how you came to know what you know. That is where the power is. I have my experience. I need yours. People speak differently when talking about what they know for themselves.

Also, I only want to hear about a religion or philosophy or principle from someone who believes it. That is the only accurate way to know what someone believes. One can't rely on their enemies to give an accurate view of someone else's beliefs. Unfortunately for many, I did get it from those who believe it, and it was still very messed up. I have heard what enemies say I supposedly believe without any of them ever asking me, so why should I believe what they say about other people? But no one gets to dictate what someone else believes, or what something means to someone else. People can only talk about their beliefs, which may or may not match someone else's. When someone comes up with something that they say someone in my church believes, they then try to insist that I believe it, or that it is somehow a doctrine of the church. It doesn't work like that. Some people know things. When they say that we are forced to believe and say all the same stuff like some cookie-cutter religion, they are speaking of themselves or they would recognize that it isn't that way and we have freedom of thought that they don't get. Only a mindless drone would assume that everyone else in the world must be a mindless drone without ever even looking. They don't look since they might find out that they are wrong. That doesn't mean that there aren't groups out there who cater to mindless drones, or that there aren't people perfectly happy being mindless drones and being told what to think at all times. We are not interested in drones. Such people fail. We are interested in people who think for themselves, learn for themselves, and are able to lift others through their knowledge and experience. We are interested in leaders, not followers, and someone is a leader when they can lead themselves as they are required to do.

There is also the problem of people outside of this religion listening to the wrong people. It is a common occurrence that someone's pastor will tell them that out writings say this and that, but the people don't EVER actually look it up to see if that is what it says. The pastors know that their unquestioning followers will never look for themselves. The idea is to instill hatred, and it is said that people condemn that which they don't understand. The other method of lying in a more subtle way is giving partial quotes, using the "…" in there where parts were edited out to change the meaning. If you change the words you can make anything say anything you want to appear, but it is still a lie. I see that frequently. Even the media articles can make a declaration in a headline, saying that it is this church that says it, and you have to get to the very last sentence in the article before they give the disclaimer that the church had actually opposed what the headline claimed the church said. But the people who write such articles know that few people will read down that far, or read anything past the headline. Therefore they get away with the lie, keeping the truth hidden where people won't look and call them out for their self-contradiction.

The refusal to look into something because of the risk of finding out things are not as a predator is trying to claim is also a narcissist tactic that I observed growing up. A case in point being my brother seeing a book on my shelf called the Encyclopedia of Suicide, psychological and sociological subjects being of interest to me since college. He had a psychology degree and had to try to show his superiority. His girlfriend was over and he had to impress her by trashing me. She saw the book and asked something about it. My brother opened on page at random which mentioned an organization involved with suicide prevention, quickly closed the book and said it is ALL just a list of organizations. He didn't look to see what was even on the rest of the page, let alone the rest of the book. He would have then had to admit he didn't know something. To deliberately look away from something is to admit that there is something there to see.

The media can be a dangerous and tricky source of information about a group. It is all too easy to create a distortion about the scapegoat minority group of the moment. How often do they point out when a crime is committed by a cis-gender heterosexual? How many of the crimes mention someone being a natural born citizen? How often do the mention that the horrible monster has a home? How often are the quite loners who don't bother anyone listed as the victims? There are some groups that they always mention, even if the crime rates of those people are well below the average.

People do believe whatever they want, and sometimes it can be very dangerous. They can believe what they want, as long as they recognize the right of others to believe what they want. We have been warned of those who persecute others for not believing what they dictate, and that is speaking of members of this church and not necessarily coming from outside. It is a problem when people are not just coming up with their own stuff and saying that the church says so, but many try to enforce their sophistries on other. That has been a source of much friction between me and others, since I have been able to stand my ground while they had no ground to stand on but what is going on in their own heads. Someone has to stand against such destructive forces, but it is mainly a church of cowards, and I stand alone among the priests for now, as I always have.

21

Enough of that stuff for now. I was able to get to Cedars-Sinai hospital and was admitted in March 2023. They did scans and of course found the extensive inflammation from me being refused treatment at Kaiser. They gave me medication, which of course helped immediately, having me symptom free again. They listened as I explained and showed them the evidence of the lies from Kaiser that were used to stop me from being treated, and Cedars-Sinai people were willing to look at actual test results, which showed that I was right all along. Testing showed that Kaiser was lying, and it doesn't take much effort to see the contradictions in the accounts from the Kaiser doctors because of all the discrepancies in every one of their claims. The doctors at Cedars-Sinai, although it took time to sort through every lie, were able to see the truth of what Kaiser was doing to me. They also worked to get me back on Thalidomide and a new medication called Skyrizi, which would be an unknown. Thalidomide has always been the effective one, the one guaranteed to get things under control. Insurance dragged their feet on approvals, but after a few months these two medications were approved. In the mean time, I would have to get by on prednisone. In March, I was on 40 mg of prednisone, which with my absorption problems, was not enough, and I was back in the hospital in April. That time they put me on 60 mg of prednisone, which was enough to keep me symptom free. I was finally back to being able to eat anything without restriction, the output dropped by half, with the corresponding increase in fluid absorption which had been proven many times to be linked to getting medication, and all food including plants were at least breaking down and changing color like they are supposed to. The inflammation markers were brought under control – further proof of the Kaiser lies and fraud.

Due to having my intake very restricted in March before getting to the hospital, I had malnutrition and dehydration. After getting out of the hospital again in April I was placed on TPN while I recover, to get me in the best shape and strength I can get to. The nutrition is important for the Skyrizi to work. I also needed my strength back, and I needed my electrolyte problem dealt with. I really only needed fluid with electrolytes.

I had been having blood clots coming out into my bag for a couple months, but that was not necessarily unusual. I bleed every year. The damage Kaiser did to me brought me to a very bad condition, and things had gone to a life threatening stage due to the damage they did. It was almost too late when I got help. Their malpractice almost had me to the point of no return. There was much damage which would have to be addressed now, very serious damage that went beyond what the inflammation markers showed. In late April, the bleeding got extreme. I then lost about ¾ of my blood by the time I got to the hospital. They put me on solumedrol and gave me around 12 units of blood before stabilizing. I would have been dead if I had got there even a little later with that rate of blood loss. Yet, it still wasn't my worst bleed ever, or even the second or third worst. I had to wait until the right time, with a bag full of blood to show and make sure that I had lost enough to be taken seriously. At other facilities doctors have been very dismissive of my massive bleedouts, not even considering such a thing possible, and telling me why I must be wrong about how much blood I lost, even with the test results available to prove how deadly the problem is. And these massive bleeds happen every so many years, with lesser bleeds every year. I was then also able to start the Skyrizi treatment and work out getting the Thalidomide, with all the hoops that have to be jumped through to get it due to the regulations. Now I am getting treated again. One bit of surprising information that came out of the May hospital visit was that my diet was superior to TPN, since I was off of my diet in the hospital but on TPN which was supposed to meet all of my needs, yet I lost 10 pound on TPN in a short time and came out in a very unnecessarily weakened state. At home I was able to get back on my diet and gain weight and strength back. My diet has always worked, as long as I am able to handle liquids at least.

Healing will take time with this treatment, but it is happening. Healing was not possible with hostile Kaiser doctors retaliating against me, causing as much harm as they could, violating their oaths to do no harm, which means nothing more than an oath means to so many other people in a predatory society. There are exceptions, and it has been difficult to get to them for treatment, and it doesn't help when other doctors are trying to stop me from getting help from them.

The moon still sets over the Pacific to tell me to stay at one with death. The birds still sing to me at midnight to tell me to live. My device keeps turning. And a campaign of terror never ends.

I'm still alive. Now where do I go from here.

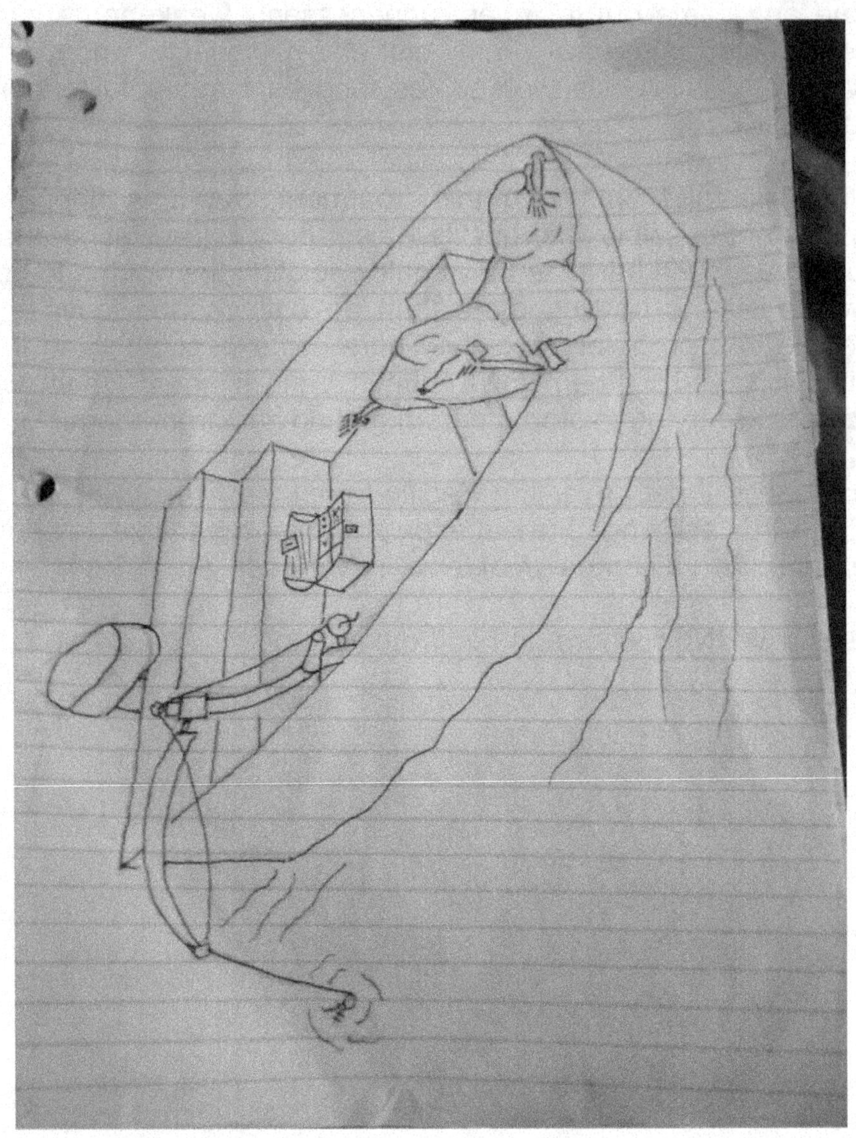

Even death needs a break sometimes

22

Some final ramblings.

There is an allegory of a young man being told to push a boulder. He did as he was advised, not knowing the purpose of the request, but trusting that the person who told him to push it knew what was right. He pushed for a long time, but the boulder never moved. After quite some time, he began to question if he had failed because the rock didn't move. The person who told him to push it then told him that he was only told to push it, not move it. The person then pointed out how strong the man had become through the effort. It was the personal development which was the point of the exercise, which was more important than the act of moving a boulder from here to there.

Some people say that the journey is more important than the end. That is close, but I would say it differently. The journey is the end, because it is only by walking a path that you get to the reward. The reward is only a dream without that path that leads there. We make the reward through our efforts.

Some refer to a disability as a "superpower". That may be somewhat of a stretch, but it is through moving on past the disability to survive which can be called a "superpower". What waits on the other side for those who overcome, and are not overcome themselves, is known only to those who have to go there. The real strength is found in continuing against the odds, when all hope is being taken away by those who claim they love you. Those who do not face opposition, who get what they want without working for it, don't know real strength, since it has never had to be used. It is no mystery why they feel threatened by someone they fail to break.

There is a reason that Native Americans considered the sickly to be shaman material.

My knowledge, what is mine which I hold inside, perspective, even the physical stuff came through the struggle with both internal and external forces of resistance. I had to bring it back with me from the brink of death. There has been no part of my life which has not been affected by this struggle, and it will never end.

Not achieving a particular set prize is not failure. You don't deserve something you are not willing to work for. If a particular set goal is not achieved, it does not mean that it "wasn't meant to be." That is just a superstition. Some things might not be attained, but that is beside the point. Circumstances can't always be changed, but that has nothing to do with what is right or wrong with walking a path. There is more to gain or lose, usually invisible things, which outsiders, society, don't see. Not attaining a "goal" does not make it wrong. Ideals are a critical part of what makes us human, and what allows us to reach higher than we have reached before. It is giving up that automatically makes something impossible and a failure, because there can never be progress in giving up. It is not wrong to hope. That is what gives us power to stretch as far as we can, that one day we may reach farther still. It is not about a score. True victory is the one the masses never see, since it happens within someone, not displayed to the world. Something may seem to be impossible, but it never actually is until one stops working toward it, and stopping is a choice. Life does not have to be forfeited, and one does not have to accept the calls to admit defeat.

The only failure is giving up. It doesn't matter if something is actually reached or not. As I said, the journey is the end. The important thing is reaching. Without reaching nothing is ever possible. Reaching makes things reachable. So never lose hope. In the darkest moments, it is a great wonder to see the foot path light up with each continued step, but it only happens as we take each step into the unseen. One must reach into the abyss until one can understand the line in the song often sung at my church which says "If we fail (death) we fail with glory.") But that is not failure. Death is not failure. Can we know the meaning of a line in another some "And if we die before our journey's through, happy day, all is well." After my death my enemies have no more power to harm me. Victory gained over them.

In the book Hagakure by Yamamoto Tsunetomo, as translated by William Scott Wilson, it says, "Although it stands to reason that a Samurai should be mindful of the Way of the Samurai, it would seem that we are all negligent.

Consequently, if someone were to ask, 'What is the Way of the Samurai?' the person who would be able to answer promptly is rare. This is because it has not been established in one's mind beforehand. From this, one's unmindfulness of the Way may be known. Negligence is an extreme thing. The Way of the Samurai is found in death. When it comes to either/or, there is only the quick choice of death. It is not particularly difficult. Be determined and advance. To say that dying without reaching one's aim is to die a dog's death is the frivolous way of sophisticates. When pressed with the choice of life or death, it is not necessary to gain one's aim. We all want to live. And in large part we make our logic according to what we like. But not having attained our aim and continuing to live is cowardice. This is a thin dangerous line. To die without gaining one's aim is to die a dog's death and fanaticism. But there is no shame in this. This is the substance of the Way of the Samurai. If by setting one's heart right every morning and evening, one is able to live as though his body were already dead, he gains freedom in the Way. His whole life will be without blame, and he will succeed in his calling." Another translation added the important line about the choice acceptance of death, that it is to see things through to the end.

So is death an enemy? It gave me what I have, it taught me all I am and know. It held my hand and walked by my side when no one else would. My closest companion. Death is considered by some, perhaps, a thief. Death doesn't take without giving, and death gives greater gifts than any person could ever give. Death understands the circle. Death is also a great teacher. Death is here to empower. Through facing death we are pushed, or push ourselves, to the limit of all we can be or do. Death guides us to make our unknown potential a reality. Death does not harm those unafraid to stare into its eyes. Death is acceptance, the acceptance society denies to those who do not conform. No one is rejected by death, but one does not have to die to have a relationship with death. It is not being dead that does the teaching. It is the journey which teaches. It is walking the path that gives the gifts with each footstep.

Once, which contemplating a problem, I had a dream explaining the nature of the issue. In this dream, there was a river to cross. There was a door on the other side of the river, and a gift was waiting on the other side of the door. There were stepping stones to use to cross the river. One could just walk right across to that door, but it wouldn't open if one tried to do it that way. There was a door at each stepping stone in the river. I had a key to the first door. I stepped on that stone and unlocked that door, and behind that door was a key to the next door. Each door had to be opened, each key had to be gained, and only the entire process could open the last door. No stone could be skipped, or things would be incomplete and knowledge would become useless distortion, and there would be no gift at the last door. It was only by walking the path right that it is realized that it was the process, each key at each door, which in the end was the gift at the end. When I got to the last door, then I understood that I already had the gift. It could be no other way. Upon waking up, it then became my job to walk that path in life. I had to see it through to the end. One can't kill themselves and expect the gift on the other side of the last door. One can't give up, or how will you get the next key? There are those who walk a very short path, just as there are those who are given a long life but never reach the gift no matter how much wasted time they have. It is how you walk the path that matters. Sidewalk or sand, it is how you walk that shows the path you are on. And, sand may have much resistance compared to walking on easy concrete, but it is in the sand that our path is marked for all to see and follow if they so choose. What death can't take from me is my life. It belongs only to me. Even if I am dead my life belongs only to me and no one else. Killing me will never make my life the property of anyone. It will always be mine, alive or dead. Therefore it is real, and it is mine. I only want what is real. All else will vanish away.

The real enemies are the living.

What I survival of the fittest? What drives evolution and progress? Isn't it adaptation? What drives adaptation? Stressors. There is no change without it. Those who don't have to face and overcome opposition don't change. Those who don't change are left behind. They are going backward in a way. Ask the beasts and be taught. Look at the many different ones and ask them why they are different. They will show you the challenges they face in their environment, and will show you the skills, mindsets, strategies, and physical powers they developed to face those challenges and oppositions, which the "normal" ones couldn't handle. Adaptation requires differences. That is, for the different who survived the murder attempts of their own mothers and grandmothers. Even the Bible tells us that it is our differences which make the whole group of us strong. What power could the body have if it consisted of only one thing – eye, hand, foot etc. and contained no other parts which are different? What happens if one of those parts decides that it is superior to all the other parts and decides that the others need to be disposed of as inferior?

A brain is certainly powerful, but it can't pump its own blood, breathe its own air, or digest the food that it runs on.

History has shown that an exclusive population invites genetic decay and disease. They help cause and become the very thing they hate. All of nature shows us that it is differences, outsiders, who keep the population strong.

Compare a human to a gorilla, and physical strength is clearly noticeably lacking in humans, even compared to other animals. How could humans become so powerful, yet be so physically weak? It is through the conditions resulting in that physical weakness that we developed even greater strength that allowed us to adapt successfully. Let's see a gorilla with great physical strength design and build a rocket and go to the moon. Humans adapted and thrived so well over natural conditions so as to even dominate and control them, even with our weak skeletons, thin skin, slow movement, lack of fangs claws thick fur/scales. We even control the destinies of the physically stronger and more dangerous animals. To give up what "weakness" has given us is to give up a part of what makes us human and to go backward. We even control our own evolutions. We have adapted the earth itself to us so well that our power even threatens the existence of us and all life. We have advanced so far that we are our own natural enemy. We have progressed so far in our conceit of being human that we have lost touch with who and what we are. In all our great learning we no longer remember our place and relation to all the other life forms. Life and the earth itself are composite beings. We are a part of nature. To destroy any part of it is to destroy a part of ourselves.

If one looks to the meaning of the Garden of Eden, one sees that one can never be happy with an illusion of happiness, one which is not earned, one never worked for, one where everything is given for nothing. It is nothing, and can never be appreciated. It is clear in the lesson that one must let go of that which is not real if one wants to obtain what is real. It is up to us to make it real. That which we can't try to reach for will never be a reality for us. It can't be given to us, only shown. We have to go there by choice, and there is no such thing as choice unless there are choices. We may have help lifting weights we can't bear on our own, we may have a guide holding our hand (the lucky ones anyway), but we must still walk, either a longer or shorter path, but walk it. No one can walk for us, and those who expect to be given, through their sense of entitlement, what is at the end of the road without going there can never know it for themselves. And those who are unwilling to go there can't tell me what is or isn't there.

The marginalized have always been the stepping stones of the supposedly superior. The "superior" only gained their lofty heights by forcing others down. What happens to the "strong", the "fittest" if we pull away, no longer fueling their egos with our blood? They will fall, and while they whine life toddlers we will see who is fittest. Those stars will fall from their bellies.

I WOULD STARE AT
A BLANK PIECE OF PAPER
EVERY DAY OF MY LIFE
IF ONE DAY I MAY DISCOVER
IT WAS NEVER BLANK AT ALL